Volume 32

PROFESSIONAL EDUCATION FOR SOCIAL WORK IN BRITAIN

PROFESSIONAL EDUCATION FOR SOCIAL WORK IN BRITAIN

An Historical Account

MARJORIE J. SMITH

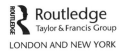

Routledge
Taylor & Francis Group

LONDON AND NEW YORK

First published in pamphlet form 1953
First published in 1965 by George Allen & Unwin Ltd

This edition first published in 2022
by Routledge
2 Park Square, Milton Park, Abingdon, Oxon OX14 4RN

and by Routledge
605 Third Avenue, New York, NY 10158

Routledge is an imprint of the Taylor & Francis Group, an informa business

British Library Cataloguing in Publication Data
A catalogue record for this book is available from the British Library

ISBN: 978-1-03-203381-5 (Set)
ISBN: 978-1-00-321681-0 (Set) (ebk)
ISBN: 978-1-03-205628-9 (Volume 32) (hbk)
ISBN: 978-1-03-205764-4 (Volume 32) (pbk)
ISBN: 978-1-00-319903-8 (Volume 32) (ebk)

DOI: 10.4324/9781003199038

Publisher's Note
The publisher has gone to great lengths to ensure the quality of this reprint but points out that some imperfections in the original copies may be apparent.

Disclaimer
The publisher has made every effort to trace copyright holders and would welcome correspondence from those they have been unable to trace.

PROFESSIONAL EDUCATION FOR SOCIAL WORK IN BRITAIN

An Historical Account

BY

MARJORIE J. SMITH

Introduction by
RICHARD M. TITMUSS

London
GEORGE ALLEN & UNWIN LTD
RUSKIN HOUSE · MUSEUM STREET

This account, by the late Professor Marjorie Smith of the British Columbia School of Social Work, tells the story of the early development of professional education for social work in Britain. In these pages she traces the work of various committees of the Charity Organisation Society on training and on social education; she touches on the contribution of great figures including Lord Avebury, Professor Alfred Marshall, Mrs Bosanquet, Sir Charles Loch and Professor Urwick; she shows the continuing struggle to establish genuine professional education through courses of integrated study and practice.

Published first by the Family Welfare Association in 1953, this study has been out of print for several years and, as it appeared originally in pamphlet form, copies have been hard to come by, even in libraries. Suggestions for a reprint came first from North America and were reinforced by requests in Britain. Thanks to the ready co-operation of the Family Welfare Association which published the original study for the Pringle Memorial Fund, the National Institute for Social Work Training is able to make available this revelation of past struggles. According to one review of the publication in its original form, it might well have been entitled 'The More Things Change the More They Remain the Same'.

First published in pamphlet form 1953
This edition first published 1965

This edition © National Institute for Social Work Training, 1965
PRINTED IN GREAT BRITAIN
in 10 point Pilgrim type
BY EAST MIDLAND PRINTING CO. LTD
BURY ST. EDMUNDS

FOREWORD

When a Fulbright research grant gave me the opportunity to study in England the origins of social casework, I did not know that I would be diverted for a time to the history of social work education. But in the process of following the development of casework ideas within the Charity Organisation Society I almost inadvertently stumbled upon the record of a tremendous effort on the part of that agency to set a standard of professional education and practice which, I do not believe, has received due attention. I found the same problems discussed and worked over by committees in 1903 as are being discussed by individuals and in committees and by conferences today. In many instances it would seem no better answers to these questions are being found than the forgotten ones of fifty years ago. One cannot help but be impressed by the calibre of people whom the Charity Organisation Society was able to interest in education for social work. Those who worked on committees and took part in conferences were among the best informed and most influential people in the country.

The reader will notice that page numbers are usually omitted in references. This was necessary because the pages of reports, papers, and records of the Charity Organisation Society were not numbered in such a way as to be useful for citation purposes.

Acknowledgements are due to Eileen Younghusband of the London School of Economics for her interest and encouragement and her direct help in relating the historical material to the current scene; and to Ben Astbury of the Family Welfare Association for his complete co-operation in making the archives of the Charity Organisation Society available. Special thanks are also due to Miss Gladys Murphy for patiently locating papers, books and reports from the library and records of the Family Welfare Association.

MARJORIE J. SMITH, 1952

CONTENTS

FOREWORD   *page* 7

INTRODUCTION BY PROFESSOR R.
    TITMUSS   11

I. Early training within the agencies   15

II. The transition to more formally organized
        training schemes   32

III. The School of Sociology   48

IV. The Amalgamation   56

V. Afterthought   66

APPENDIX

I. a. *The Training of Volunteers*, Mrs. Dunn
        Gardner, 1894   69

   b. *Extracts from the First Report of the Com-
        mittee on Training*, 1898   79

   c. *Methods of Training*, Helen Bosanquet,
        1900   85

II. *Economic Teaching at the Universities in
    Relation to Public Well-being*, Professor A.
    Marshall, 1902   93

III. *Extracts from the Confidential Report of the
     Social Education Committee*, 1903   103

INTRODUCTION

From time to time it is necessary to remind our students (and ourselves) that specialization in knowledge – the study of a subject or branch of learning deeply and thoroughly – does not imply the neglect of all other subjects. This is pre-eminently true of the social sciences, for those who have permanently enriched our knowledge of the working of society have not been specialists in any narrow or technical sense. Their special learning has been cultivated within a broad field of study; they have acquired an approach which sees and relates the parts to the whole. Today, as knowledge expands and is increasingly subdivided, the separated parts tend to get smaller in range as study is pushed ever deeper, and the connecting threads weaken as each part achieves separate independence in the commonwealth of learning. Knowledge grows, but the threat to unitary understanding increases.

In social work, as in medicine, two fields of applied knowledge which above all others demand the general and the special practitioner for the understanding and care of the individual in trouble, the dangers of specialization are considerable. We can do more; we can understand and help more; but we can also harm more. It is a wholesome sign that since the end of the Second World War these dangers to social work (and, again, to medicine) have received more recognition. What, in particular, is serious for the future well-being of social work is specialization in function and specialization at the wrong time in the processes of learning. Together, these can easily lead to a widening in the gulf between thought and action; between academic study and practical life. The Universities, concerned as they are with what is clumsily called the 'pre-vocational education' of those entering social work and other professions, cannot remain aloof.

It is one of the fundamental purposes of the University to build bridges – not dismantle them – as Alfred Marshall pointed out exactly 50 years ago when he addressed the Committee on Social Education convened by the Charity Organisation Society. English action, he said, had been largely separated from English thought and he looked (as did the Webbs) to the younger and then less respectable subjects of economics and political science to remedy this fault. One practical step which followed from this movement of ideas was significant for the future of social work : in 1912 the London School of Economics itself proposed to the Charity Organisation Society that it should take over the educational functions of the London School of Sociology in relation to the education of social workers. A new Department of Social Science and Administration was formed, the success of which would depend, said the Charity Organisation Society, 'on the Director having been himself trained in the practical duties of case work'.

It is to Professor Marjorie Smith, an American citizen, of the University of British Columbia, that we are indebted for reminding us of this not unimportant episode in the history of social work in Britain, and of the consequences, in theory and practice, which have flowed from these early developments. But she has done more than that; in this historical study she has described and interpreted the ferment of thought and inquiry at the beginning of the century into the problems of social work education and practice inspired and stimulated, as it was, by the Charity Organisation Society in London. The fact that she found the same problems of specialization and of relating theory and practice being discussed and worked over by committees in 1903 as are being discussed today is a reflection of neglected research into the origins and development of social work in Britain. This failing adds point to the warnings that are implicit in Professor Smith's study; once again we are reminded, clearly and forcibly, that social work education needs re-thinking in terms of fundamental principles.

In welcoming the publication of this study by the Family Welfare Association it gives me an opportunity to express, on behalf of the staff of the Department, our gratitude for all that Professor Smith contributed in research and teaching during her stay of a year in the Department. Professor Smith helped with many bridges, transcontinental and domestic, and we are glad that the award of a Fulbright Research Grant made all this possible.

RICHARD M. TITMUSS, 1952

CHAPTER I

EARLY TRAINING WITHIN
THE AGENCIES

THE history of social work in Britain reveals that much more was done about the training of social workers than is generally known. By 1896, a co-operative scheme of training through lectures and practical work had been established. Fifty years ago the Charity Organisation Society urged the founding of a professional school of social work on a university level and such an institution came into being in 1903. Subsequently, from time to time, when the hopes for widespread professional education schemes were not fulfilled, the Charity Organisation Society tried to direct the attention of the public to the need for professional education. The training of the practitioner was not developed within the social science departments of universities and has remained for the most part under the sponsorship of social agencies and government departments except during the 1903-12 period when the independent School of Sociology was in existence. The need for general professional education for social work, however, was made clear, not only in 1903, but in 1919 and again in 1947.

The current situation with its numbers of separate, specialized courses designed to train the worker for vocational fields; the immobility of such persons; and the ever-present shortage of qualified people again forces to the front the problem of social work education. In relation to this, the thoughts and plans of the pioneers of the past are particularly relevant. Many of their statements sound startlingly modern, in many instances without even translation into current terminology, and provide the answers to questions still being asked.

The first ideas about training social workers came naturally from the development of several activities, including the work of Octavia Hill, who, on organizing and carrying out her plan of rent collecting (begun in 1864), found it necessary to enlist the help of others when she could not do all the work herself. She, personally, began to teach new recruits her methods of helping the poor when it became obvious that some kind of apprenticeship training was essential. As time went on people came from distant places to be trained and the work expanded to the point where something more elaborate had to be arranged. During the same period of time the Women's University Settlement in Southwark was training its new volunteers, and it was Miss Margaret Sewell, the Warden, who first saw and acted upon the possibility of teaching the new workers partially through the medium of group instruction in lectures and classes. Miss Hill and Miss Sewell joined forces about 1890, and volunteers, as well as paid employees, were trained for both the Settlement and the rent-collecting plan through lectures at the Settlement and by practical work in both settings.

During the same years, the Charity Organisation Society, through its district committees, was also training workers by setting them to tasks in the practical work of the district offices. By 1895, the business of training volunteer workers had become an important part of the work of the district committees.

During this early period there were three papers which stand out as historic documents. The first was read to the Charity Organisation Society by Mrs Dunn Gardner, November 26, 1894, on the subject of the training of volunteers. The second was the first report of the Committee on Training, adopted by the Council of the Charity Organisation

Society in December, 1898; and the third was a paper by Helen Bosanquet read to the Society in 1900.

Mrs Gardner's paper,[1] being the earliest available document on the training of the social worker, is worthy of special attention. It sums up the need for training and suggests methods for practical work which in many ways are in line with modern thinking. Mrs Gardner stated in 1894 a problem which still calls for attention at times. She makes it clear that a student is not to be considered an asset for getting work done, but rather as a learner who must be taught:

> We must at once dismiss from our minds the idea that workers are to be trained only with a view to their being useful to their trainers. Often when the subject of volunteers is being discussed I have heard people say, 'Oh, I would so much rather do the work myself!' Of course they would – it would take half the time, and less than half the trouble, of getting someone else to do it – but the result attained would be quite different.

Mrs Gardner's suggestions about the proper way to introduce new workers to the field are also of interest and useful in current situations:

> Now, I should like to lay special stress on two points. One is that the first thing to do with new workers is to *interest* them: if we fail to do this, I think we shall not get far in training them. And the second point to which I want to draw attention goes hand in hand with the first, and it is that you must make all workers – old as well as new, for the matter of that – feel their own *responsibility*. It is useless to expect anyone to go on regularly doing anything unless he feels that it makes

[1] *C.O.S. Occasional Papers*—First Series. No. 46. Reprinted from *Charity Organisation Review*, January, 1895.

some difference to somebody whether he does it or not. No doubt his attendance must often involve considerable personal inconvenience, and, if he finds that things go on equally well, whether he does or does not keep his engagements, it is only natural that he should stay away when it is difficult for him to come – but once let him be sure that inconvenience or delay, or suffering, will follow on his failing to do what he has undertaken, and you will find he is very unlikely to let anything stand in the way of his work.

The Secretary has generally from the very first two courses open to him. Probably there is some bit of work at the office which is standing over till it can get taken in hand. The new worker may have this bit of work explained to him, and may be set down to carry it on. If he happens to take to it, well and good; if not, why then he will soon leave off coming to the office, and the same bit of work will be ready to hand to choke off the next energetic aspirant after employment. . . . Or instead of instructing him in this special bit of work, the Secretary may, to the best of his ability, try to train the newcomer, not for any special work, but for work itself; may, in fact, teach him not to make the head of the pin, or the point of the pin, but the whole article.

Mrs Gardner's emphasis on teaching the 'whole' to the learner rather than giving him a bit of detailed instruction about specific errands is merely good educational method, and it is what we recognize today as necessary in the education of social workers. Students must be taught not only specific narrow technical activities but must learn to know the part in relation to the whole. The individual's need in relation to community, the bearing of administration on resources available to assist the individual, the whole situation and all its ramifications.

The need for supervision and for a general orientation to the office are clearly outlined by Mrs Gardner:

Of course, all this involves a great deal of inspection, and calls for constant patience and tact on the part of the Secretary (for instance, he will often find the letter about the Notice B Committee case, of the boy Jones, carefully put away in the Pension box, on the case of widow Jones), but ill results from such mistakes are easily guarded against by proper supervision. In letter writing it may be a long time before any letter written by a new-comer can be sent out, and often the Secretary will have to spend part of his afternoon in rewriting the letters produced by volunteers in the morning. But this only lasts for a time, a time varying in length with each worker; for let us always remember that our workers have quite as varied natures as our applicants, and require to be dealt with in quite as varied a manner. . . . When the new worker has seen something of all that is being done at a C.O.S. office he is in a position to decide for what branch of the work he feels most interested and is most suited.

Mrs Gardner states the necessity for learners to read and suggests that each office add to the few books it already has so that there would be a real library relating directly to the work. Also she emphasizes the need to train more workers than were needed for the Charity Organisation Society work and that the organization had responsibility to supply train-ing for many others if the general condition of the poor were to be improved.

The importance of training was further emphasized in the 28th Annual Report of the Charity Organisation Society, covering the year 1895-96:[2]

[2] *Twenty-Eighth Annual Report of the Charity Organisation Society*, March 12, 1897.

'Training' or the education of the worker, is assuming every year a more prominent place in the work of the Society. . . . Consequently to train volunteers is now the recognized function of many Committees. There are, perhaps, four grades of these learners. Some come out of a kind of philanthropic curiosity. They do not master the art of charity, even pretend to do so. This work is hard, and, if well done, it is a tax alike on energy and intelligence. But they will not make the required effort, and they quickly turn to other things.

Another group is anxious to learn, and have all the ability necessary for simple and straightforward almoner-ship. They will learn what to avoid and they will culti-vate a new dutifulness in charity. They will never become mere tract distributors. They will always think it wrong to do what has sometimes been said to be necessary and inevitable – give a ticket or trifle when they visit the poor, as a kind of payment for admission. They are not people who visit a Charity Organisation Committee for occupation only. They are bona-fide doers.

Another group consists of those who, before they begin work in connection with clergy or ministers or associa-tions, come to learn what the Society's methods are. It takes two to co-operate, as it is said to take two to make a quarrel. These persons are the future co-operators with the Charity Organisation Committees. Unless they be trained, and understand the methods of charity and accept its principles, they will bar progress instead of advancing it. . . . Educated, they are the natural allies of Charity Organisation. Untrained, they will unwittingly be its opponents. There is, therefore, no question of the claim of this group of workers upon the good offices of the Society. No part of its organization is more important than that which is engaged in their education. Happily, the number of those who come to the Society with a view to working elsewhere ultimately is on the increase.

The last group is relatively small. It consists of those who will continue to work for the Society, and may become its leaders, as hon. secretaries, chairmen, or members of Committee. On them principally the well-being of the Society must depend.

This statement outlines the training needs for various levels of work: (1) those who were not particularly serious in their interest, (2) those who were to become good workers, (3) those who would be working in other fields than the Charity Organisation Society, and (4) those who were to fill the top ranks of the Society. Most interesting, perhaps, is the acceptance of responsibility for training those in the third group, and although the reason given is a self-interest one, it does indicate an understanding of the broader needs of the field and that training could be given for more than the specific work of one agency.

The 28th Annual Report also indicates that a Joint Lectures Committee had been organized in the autumn of 1896 consisting of representatives of the Women's University Settlement in Southwark, the National Union of Women Workers, and the Charity Organisation Society. The report explains:

> Miss Sewell, the Warden of the Women's University Settlement, and Miss Miranda Hill delivered the first course of lectures on charity and almsgiving, which were very well attended. And this spring Miss Sophia Lonsdale and Miss Bannatyne deliver a second course on the Poor Law. Other lectures are also being given by Miss Sharpley at Bethnal Green and Chelsea. In all these lectures stress is laid on the practical side of charitable work, numerous instances are cited, and the application of the principles of charity explained.

This can be considered the first organized attempt to train

social workers generally for the field, placing an emphasis upon teaching theoretical methods combined with practical work in agencies.

The problem of employed district secretaries also concerned the Council of the Charity Organisation Society during this year. Much earlier (1883) the Society had accepted the principle of employed secretaries, in contrast to all voluntary workers, but apparently there had been some objection to it. It was thought that such workers would be likely to supersede and to lessen the number or the need for voluntary workers. A special committee was appointed in 1896 which brought in a number of resolutions subsequently adopted by the Council in 1897. These resolutions included one for the formation of a Committee on Training which was to study the best practical method of in-service training for paid and voluntary workers within the Society.

In the 29th Annual Report (1896-97) the following is noted:

Training

The *Committee on Training*, referred to in the fifth resolution, has since been appointed, and arrangements have been made for the attendance of District Secretaries on probation at lectures, and for their paying visits to institutions; and opportunities are afforded both to those who may become Honorary Secretaries and to Secretaries on probation to come for a time to the Central Office and there obtain an insight into the general work of the Society.

This report also indicates that the Joint Lectures Committee had appointed Miss M. McN. Sharpley as a paid lecturer who, with others, delivered a series of lectures. It is interesting and valuable to consider the 'curriculum' arranged by the Joint Committee. A series of lectures were set up for a two-year period from the Autumn of 1896 to the Spring of 1898. There is a continuity and visible integration of content much in line with modern professional social work education. Miss Sewell, of the University Women's Settlement, headed the programme with four lectures on 'The Scope of Charitable Work', followed by four lectures from Miss Miranda Hill (sister of Octavia) on 'The Family and Character', 'Personal Work', 'Co-operation in Charity', 'Thoroughness'. Put into modern language it would seem that in the Autumn the students had a course in 'the field of social work' followed by a course in 'principles and methods'.

In the Spring, Miss Sophia Lonsdale gave four lectures on the history of the English Poor Law, followed by Miss Bannatyne with four lectures on 'The Care of Women and Children Under the Poor Law'. The students had, therefore, added to their previous term's work the content of State relief and social services for certain groups under special disability.

In the following Autumn, Mrs Bosanquet gave four lectures on 'The Standard of Life' and Mr Blandford four on 'The Co-operative Movement'. These courses were obviously an attempt to broaden the students' interest in social economic questions. In the Spring of 1898 the entire time was devoted to material relating to children. First came four lectures from Mr Chance (later Sir William Chance) on 'Education, Training, and Care of Children Under the Poor Law', followed by four single lectures as follows: the Rev Brooke Lambert on 'Industrial and Reformatory Schools'; Miss Eve on 'Care and Education of Children in Industrial Schools in Connection with the School Board'; Dr Francis Warner on 'Children Who Require Special Care and Training'; and Mr W. M. Acworth on 'Children Under the Metropolitan Asylums Board'.

Taken as a whole, this programme of lectures, combined with practical work, would have provided a balanced introduction to the field. Considering that there were no State social services other than Poor Law Relief and certain special institutions, one must come to the conclusion that the content was fairly comprehensive. When one remembers, also, the results of the Curtis Committee study in 1946, the emphasis placed on child care by these pioneers of fifty years before was entirely justified.

In addition to the Central London organized lectures, a number of the same ones were given in some outlying districts of London and in the provinces. The following year there was added to the series a number of lectures on 'Medical Relief', including topics relating to medical charities, the hospital, the lunatic asylum, district nursing, the poor-law infirmary, sick insurance, and others. Miss Sharpley, the paid lecturer, devoted her time to the lectures on Principles and Methods, and volunteer and honorary lecturers presented knowledge and content of various social services and problems according to their interests and experience.[3]

The fact, which is borne out by later experience, that education for social work has always operated on scanty funds, is brought home by the 30th Annual Report of the Council as it goes on to say:

A word should be added as to the finance. Mrs G. F. Hill is the Hon. Secretary of the Lectures Committee. To her the Council are very greatly indebted for the great care and consideration with which she has arranged the various courses. Miss Powell is the Hon. Treasurer of the Committee. Miss Sharpley's salary is £150 a year. Towards this the Council have paid £37 10s in the present financial year. The Lectures Committee have received for the same purpose a promise of £100 from an anonymous donor, and part of the salary will probably be met

[3] *Thirtieth Annual Report of the Charity Organisation Society*, March 6, 1899.

by a grant made on behalf of the Women's University Settlement, and by the proceeds of the Lectures. The Lectures Committee publishes a separate report and accounts.

From the same report, it is of interest to note that the Committee and those concerned with training progressed in their thinking about methods of teaching, and moved from the idea of lectures only to classes involving short talks and discussions as an additional means:

> In the Autumn a very well attended Conference was held to consider the best means of providing lectures for District Visitors or Local Workers. The result has been that the Lectures Committee have agreed to endeavour to arrange for short talks and discussions with such workers on special subjects or on points of difficulty.

Present day social work education relies on three methods: Lectures for certain content; discussion classes and groups, particularly for professional technical material; and individual supervision or teaching in practical work and research. It would seem that the Joint Lectures Committee in 1898 had begun to use all these ways of training and teaching.

The 'Special Committee on Training' referred to in the 29th Annual Report of the Council of the Charity Organisation Society (see page 7) was appointed on the 28th day of June, 1897. The Committee consisted of: Mr W. A. Bailward, Miss Bruce, Mr A. H. Paterson, Miss M. Sewell, Mr R. Sharpe, Mr H. V. Toynbee, Mr A. Wedgwood, Mr H. Woollcombe. They met eleven times and held a conference on the subject of training before submitting their first report which was adopted by the Council on December 12, 1898.[4]

[4] 'First Report of the Committee on Training', C.O.S. *Occasional Papers* – Second Series – No. 11.

The Committee in its report outlined the problem it had been given, that is, the training of executive members of the Society. They defined in a sense what these workers should be trained for, and in so doing made clear the main objectives or principles of the Society:

> The general impression derived from the discussion at the Conference already alluded to was that there still prevails amongst some of the executive members of District Committees a want of grasp of the principles for which the Society exists, and a want of enthusiasm for their fulfilment. There was general agreement, for instance, amongst those who attended the Conference, that almost all those who join the Society do so in the first instance for the sake of its relief work, and that many never get beyond that stage. 'General business' involving the discussion of principles, aroused only a languid interest at District Committees, and the discussion was as a rule confined to one or two members of the Committee. This want of interest in principles was not confined to the new recruits only, but extended itself even to those who had been working for the Society for a considerable period.
>
> The great development of the case-work of the Society of late years has evidently become a new danger in this respect. It has naturally a more concrete and direct personal interest than the advocacy of principles, and, as all experience shows, may easily monopolize the whole time and attention of a band of workers necessarily limited. The question does not, of course, come within the scope of the inquiry of this Committee except in so far as the subject of training is concerned, and therefore the Committee would merely emphasize in passing the essential importance of inculcating principles as early as possible in the education of a learner, of impressing upon him that case-work is mainly to be used as a means

of organization, and that the 'improvement of the condition of the poor' as a whole is a much nobler and more far-reaching object than the relief of a certain number of cases of distress.

It is obvious from this statement that the Committee thought the training should be properly directed towards teaching principles and methods of organization rather than methods of dealing with individual need.

The Report continues at some length to suggest and outline actual ways of teaching, drawing heavily on Mrs Gardner's earlier paper, and concludes with a rather far-reaching statement:

In conclusion, the Training Committee feel that, as they have already indicated, there is no royal road to training, and their hope for the future is rather based upon the wider interest in the subject which is now being manifested than upon any suggestion which they or anyone else can supply. They believe that the Society as a training Society is as yet in its infancy, and that it is capable of almost boundless development. They believe that if the educational functions of the Society were more fully recognized by the public it would lead to a much wider appreciation of its work and expansion of its influence. They would like to see in the Society the nucleus of a future university for the study of social science, in which all those who undertake philanthropic work should desire to graduate.

In an appendix, the Committee lists recommended books as follows:

'The Occasional Papers' (C.O.S.).
'Rich and Poor' : Mrs Bosanquet.

'How to Help Cases of Distress' (The Handbook of the
C.O.S.).
'Our Common Land' : Miss Octavia Hill.
'Charity Organisation' : Mr C. S. Loch.
'Capital, Trade, Labour, and the Outlook' : Miss Benson.

Two years later, Mrs Bosanquet gave a paper on *Methods
of Training*[5] which immediately took the classical position
held by Mrs Gardner's paper of six years before.

Mrs Bosanquet emphasized, first, the importance of the
learner being a student and not merely immersed in work.
She objected to the 'sink or swim' method of introducing
the new worker to the field, and stated the beginner 'should
be definitely a student, and not an additional office boy.
That does not mean, of course, that he is never to do anything useful; but it does mean that he is to approach the
work from an entirely different point of view . . . we
tend to welcome the active, energetic person who likes
running about the district on his bicycle and enjoys nothing
so much as making a dozen disconnected inquiries on a
dozen different cases which just need completing for committee. Compared with him the person who is always raising difficulties and asking explanations is very troublesome,
and hardly less so the person who sits for hours puzzling
himself and others over one set of case-papers.' She goes
on to say in her own unique way: 'But thinking is not
always a waste of time; and the student who is neither
thinking nor asking questions may do an immense amount
of miscellaneous work without getting much further in
understanding.'

Mrs Bosanquet spends some time on resistance to learning. She states that most difficult to deal with is the prejudice against reading or learning of any kind. ' "There is too
much real work to be done," one will say; "I have no time

[5] Helen Bosanquet, 'Methods of Training' in *C.O.S. Occasional
Papers* – Third Series – No. 3.

for your books and theories." ' She adds that a milder form of this same prejudice is evidenced in 'the student who wants to devote himself to one branch of work without knowing anything of others. "I don't want to read about the poor law," he will explain, "it's not the kind of work that I care about." But though this is an age of specialization, the student must be made to see that he cannot afford to neglect any of the influences affecting the lives in which he is interested: that specialization indeed means learning more, not less. *A man is not a specialist because he knows only one thing, but because he knows one thing better than others.*'[6]

This statement about specialization could bear some careful consideration in the light of today's 'over-specialization' in the training of social workers.[7] What had been achieved more recently is not specialization but rather a break-up of a larger skill into bits and pieces much as the old handicraft skills have been broken up to achieve factory production on a mass basis. The inappropriateness of this division of social skill and method applied to the treatment of human problems is becoming more apparent every day.

Broad outlines of training methods were discussed by Mrs Bosanquet. First, she states, the student must have his aims or objectives defined. 'The student must be taught what the good is that he wishes to do, before he can be taught how to do it.' In the second place he must be taught how to achieve his aims, and this knowledge will come from a study of the actual experience of others, from reading case-papers and the history of poor law and other methods. Mrs Bosanquet places first, the learning of principles, attitudes, and social philosophy, and secondly, on that base, the learning of skills, and in so doing has stated the modern concept of social work education. In her paper, she

[6] Italics are the writer's.
[7] See: E. L. Younghusband, *Social Work in Britain* (Edinburgh, 1951).

describes how the student can learn about the community by studying a particular district and all the forces at work in that district; and she spends some time on the casework method itself: 'Perhaps the principle on which I should like to lay most stress with reference to training in casework, is that we keep the student from falling into anything like conventionality. Conventional ways of classifying cases, conventional modes of help, conventional rules for making inquiries, all are dangerous, and especially dangerous in our work. It is comparatively easy to learn the little list of categories: *Not likely to benefit, Left to Clergy, Poor Law case, Necessary information refused,* and to class our case under it; what is more important and difficult is to learn how to keep it out of one of these classes, and this requires an insight to which every case is unique and individual.' This is a clear statement of the fundamental casework principle of individualization of human problems. The paper ends in expression of the idea of the dual role of the social worker:

> We talk a great deal in our work about the necessity of plans. Really the student has to learn to combine two plans – the one of helping the individual case, the other of raising the district to which it belongs. It is less difficult than it seems at first, for the contradiction which sometimes appears between the two is only apparent, or at most temporary. Moreover, it is a difficulty which all artists have to solve, that of developing both the part and the whole without sacrificing either, in order to attain harmony. I say all artists, for there is always something of the artist about the true philanthropist, and the harmony of life which he aims at creating is hardly less important than that of the painter, the poet, or musician.

This double role of the social worker has been forgotten again and again in the last fifty years. At times it has looked

as though the emphasis placed on reform and mass improvement by some people is totally incompatible with the bias
of others towards method and skill, and that those who are
primarily interested in technique cannot be reconciled with
those whose aims are turned toward organization and
administration. It has remained for such leaders as Mrs
Bosanquet, and Porter Lee,[8] many years later in America,
to point out this double-headed aim and objective which
must, of necessity, influence the kind of training and education provided for social workers.

[8] Porter Lee, *Social Work as Cause and Function* (New York, 1937).

CHAPTER II

THE TRANSITION TO MORE FORMALLY
ORGANIZED TRAINING SCHEMES

THE work of the Joint Lectures Committee continued for
another three years, i.e. until the Committee was dissolved
in July of 1901. Lectures were continued on similar lines as
in the first two years with subjects added as the social service scene shifted and changed. One cannot help but notice
the flexibility of the Committee in changing the content
of lectures as the field changed and as new developments
arose. The core of the course remained: (1) 'Principles and
Methods', (2) 'Charitable work', and (3) 'The English Poor
Laws'. Housing was a new subject, as was the relation
between 'poor law and charity' which would be a logical
addition because of the agitation for poor law reform during
the period.

The dissolution of the Joint Lectures Committee came
about naturally enough through the activities and development of the 'Special Committee on Training'. The Special
Committee of the Council of the Charity Organisation
Society was, as we have seen, established primarily to study
means of improving the practical training of workers in the
district offices and the specific training needed by those who
would be working in the Charity Organisation Society itself.
It is interesting to note that the Course as arranged by the
Joint Lectures Committee was always referred to as 'Lectures and Education' and that which was the concern of
the Special Committee was called 'training'. There is reason
behind this distinction and it reflects certain concepts which

have troubled the social work educators of more recent times. The distinction between professional education and mere technical or specific training is clear and those who were working with the problem at the beginning of the 20th Century were making a distinction between that which was considered educational and that which was purely technical. The error lay in not seeing that professional education for social work, like all professional education, necessarily includes certain technical study related to theory or based upon theoretical knowledge. Although it was apparent to the earlier educators that both theoretical instruction and practical training were necessary in the education of social workers, they could not see how the two could be logically interwoven. They were confused in this issue primarily because technical methods had not as yet been developed to the point at which they could be recognized as an academically acceptable and teachable content.

In an attempt to dissolve this conflict the Charity Organisation Society planned an extension of the system of lectures previously arranged by the Joint Lectures Committee. Under a section of the 33rd Annual Report[1] of the Charity Organisation Society headed 'Social Education' the story is told of a circular issued in the Autumn of 1901 to 'some members of the Universities and others interested in economic and social work, asking them to become members of a General Committee for the purpose, if they approved of the proposed scheme'. Apparently the response was favourable because many University professors' names appear as members of the Committee. The scheme 'suggested an alliance . . . between the professors at Universities and Colleges, and members of Settlements and of Charity Organisation Societies' for the purpose of social education. It was proposed that in towns where there was a

[1] *Thirty-third Annual Report of the Charity Organisation Society,* March 19, 1902.

University or College a Committee be established and that lectures and practical work be arranged.

In centres where there was no University, the Committees should be formed and some plan of co-operative effort be worked out. 'In this way it is hoped sufficient scope will be given to the two elements necessary to social education – on the one hand, a knowledge of theory and history, and on the other actual observation and personal experience.'

The local Committees were to be federated for purposes of mutual help and were to have representation on the enlarged central committee in London.

The circular outlined the plan of lectures in this way :

> To make the Lectures useful, it would be necessary that in conjunction with them, at Settlements and in the Charity Organisation Committees, positive work should be undertaken under definite guidance, so that the actual difficulties of social and economic questions may be realized in relation to the lives and circumstances of those in want or distress. The true bearing of various methods and opinions on the needs and treatment of individuals and families, on the administration of poor relief, and on more general questions, such as labour and the condition of the labouring classes, education, 'housing', and sanitation, would thus be brought to light and emphasized.
>
> It is desired to make the Lectures of use to persons undertaking voluntary or paid service, such as clergymen or ministers in connection with eleemosynary work, medical men in connection with medical relief, school managers, Poor Law Guardians and Relieving Officers, trustees of endowed charities, members or officers of charitable societies, and district visitors.
>
> It is proposed to include in the Lectures courses on the history of Charity, Social Economics and Statistics, Institutional administration, the administration of relief

in its various branches, and on many of the proposals for social progress. The classes and courses will be systematic, and as far as possible carried on in conjunction with definite practical work. It is intended also to issue from time to time publications, reprints, etc., that may be of service in connection with the courses of Lectures and classes.

This scheme for co-operation between universities and agencies is a fairly complete plan for professional education, judged by modern standards, including an association of schools and the producing and publishing of professional literature for teaching purposes. Mr Loch (later Sir Chas. Loch), General Secretary of the Charity Organisation Society, was the leader in this development and he was the first person to propose that the Universities should become responsible for the education of social workers. It was out of this plan that the School of Social Science at Liverpool was established in 1904 through a co-operative arrangement among the University, the Victoria Settlement for Women and the Liverpool Central Relief and Charity Organisation Society.[2] Other similar arrangements quickly followed.

The final report of the Joint Lectures Committee which is appended to the 33rd Annual Report of the Charity Organisation Society, gives an account of what happened in the summer of 1901 in reference to the dissolution of the Committee. Apparently the Women's University Settlement withdrew from the Joint Committee upon the proposal to extend the work to centres outside London. Their Articles of Association confined their work to London and they did not feel justified in being part of a committee acting in a larger area. 'It was with the greatest regret that the Joint Committee found itself obliged to accept this decision as

[2] See: Elizabeth Macadam, *The Social Servant in the Making*, p. 23. George Allen & Unwin, Ltd, London, 1946.

final, and acquiesce on the loss of the help of the body to which the lecture scheme owed its origin.'[3]

The only practical course left was for the Committee to become a new special committee of the Council of the Charity Organisation Society. The original members were now constituted as the 'Committee on Social Education', and the official connection with the National Union of Women Workers was severed.

Work was immediately begun to extend the training plan. Lectures were arranged for London as before and for Birmingham and preliminary lectures were given at Glasgow.

In October, 1902, a conference was called of the members of the Social Education Committee, and others who might be interested were invited to participate. The obvious intent was to discuss the problem of University teaching of the social sciences. Lord Avebury, who presided, opened the proceedings with some statements regarding the current discussions in Parliament on the Education Bill. He spoke of the lack of attention given to educational theory. 'He deprecated too early specialization, and contended that up to the age of sixteen and seventeen their efforts should be directed to laying a solid foundation of general knowledge and culture, including more science and modern languages . . . and the scientific teaching should include economic theory, which had been unwisely depreciated.'[4]

Professor A. Marshall was called upon to give the opening paper on 'Economic Teaching at the Universities in Relation to Public Well-being'. He outlined the changing economic and social conditions in the world which called for leaders who were trained, not only in realistic technical matters, but who had had the opportunity for the broader develop-

[3] *Thirty-third Annual Report of the Charity Organisation Society.* March 19, 1902.
[4] *Charity Organisation Review*, January, 1903.

ment of imaginative powers which only the University could give.

'Every science,' he stated, 'requires and trains in various degrees these three faculties – perception, imagination, reason: the use of these constitutes the centre of the intellectual life of every University. But perhaps there is no science which requires all three in more even proportions than economics; none, therefore, which more properly is of University rank. And, in addition, economic studies train the sympathies together with the intellect. This task, which truly belongs to the University, is most excellently performed in its social life, but not equally well in its studies.' His charge that the Universities must recognize their responsibility for teaching realistic action as well as thought concluded with this statement:

> Greek thought and Greek action, political and social, were indissolubly welded together. But English action has been largely separated from English thought. This did, indeed, relatively little harm while English action was chiefly given to bringing into subjection uncivilized races beyond the oceans, and to developing industries which were strong but insular and crude. But it is doing untold harm now that the Western world is in effect one, now that some other nations are in certain respects marching quicker and are more alert than we, and now that social and economic problems are becoming every day more urgent, partly because our growing wealth and knowledge is every day increasing our responsibilities. All hail, then, to the Committee on Social Education, which is to combine social thought and action in a modern temper, but in due subordination to the great Greek doctrine that the Ideal is that which is most truly Real!

In the discussion which followed, a number of University representatives spoke, a few in favour of the proposals but a number objected to the idea of combining practical work with university education. Professor Chapman, of Owen's College, Manchester, put it in this fashion:

'The University must, of course, be impartial in its teaching. Any attempt to superimpose principles upon a groundwork of general education would tend to make partisans without independent thought and convictions. The part of the University was to inform and train the student's mind and to give him the power of judgment. Principles of action must be acquired elsewhere.'

A member of the Committee, Mr Medd, made a forthright statement in that 'he thought that they would be wiser to keep clear of the Universities, which in social questions were amateurish and academic, and were designed to produce graduates. They wanted something more like the Amsterdam School of Social Work, combining study of theory with actual work. He suggested a two-year course as a minimum, with a third year at the student's option.'

The result of the discussion was a resolution to create a Trust which would provide lectures and teaching combined, if possible, with practical work under definite guidance. Further resolutions were passed calling on the Executive Committee of the Committee on Social Education to prepare a report making suggestions as to how the instruction offered by the universities in moral science, history, and economics could best be used in connection with the work of the proposed Trust and also to prepare a suggested syllabus of lectures and teaching. These resolutions were discussed and adopted by the Council of the Charity Organisation Society on November 10, 1902.

The Conference of the Social Education Committee obviously arrived at a definite point of view. First, it agreed that it was necessary for social workers and others who worked in public business to be educated *and* trained, that they must have theoretical and practical work. Second, the conference framed, but did not attempt to solve, the problem of the relationship of the universities to this newer idea of education for public service. The resolution for the establishment of a Trust for the purpose of providing the desired teaching indicates their decision that the work must be done by an organization outside, or at least independent of, the universities.

The report called for from the Executive Committee was submitted as a private and confidential document for consideration by the Council on June 8, 1903.[5] It was a comprehensive statement including a summary of the teaching then being done in the universities, suggested courses of lectures, teaching and 'positive' work for students, with added suggestions of courses for students who intended to enter ministerial work, those engaged or likely to be engaged in Poor Law relief, and those in charity work either volunteer or paid. The report is worth considering in detail. Its first section is a survey of the various lectures then given in the universities. It pointed out that the programme offered by the London School of Economics included much that was important, and the report states that it had been suggested that the Social Education Committee attach its work to that School. The Committee expressed its disapproval of this suggestion in these words :

A consideration of the two-year course proposed below will show that it is distinctive and materially different from the courses provided at the School of Economics. It is related all through to social life and practical administration, with which the lectures and reading are closely linked, and on which they are for the most part dependent. Also the social and ethical side of the teaching which is apparent in the two-year course, and to which

[5] *Minutes of the Council*, Charity Organisation Society, June, 1903.

yet larger scope might indeed be given, as essential to a right treatment of social problems, is almost wholly wanting in the courses provided by the School of Economics. Lastly, the tone and character of that institution is marked, and alike in its inception and in the public estimation of its work and position it has been associated conspicuously with one school of thought.

Laying aside the matter of the particular school of thought which controlled the London School of Economics, the Committee, whether they realized or not, were indicating there was still a difference in the kind of education they wanted for social workers from that available in the regular academic work of the universities. This thinking was further amplified in the Committee's summary statement of the section devoted to a survey of university courses :

To sum up, then, as to the means of 'teaching Social Science and Economics, with special reference to social obligation and administration' these various curricula (good and useful as they are in many ways) appear to have no sufficiently practical connection with social problems and the actual conditions of life as they come to light and are dealt with in administration; and in consequence, judged from the standpoint of social science and obligation, they would seem likely to produce comparatively small results, or even, in some degree, results that may be harmful. They may produce comparatively small results, for the question discussed in connection with them may rouse but little interest, if they are considered apart from practical issues and needs and their real meaning is not understood, while the student is tempted to regard them only as part of the book-work incidental to examinations and progress through life. On the other hand these curricula may produce results that may in some degree be even harmful. They may lead to ill-balanced and ill-proportioned conceptions of society, which may prove very misleading and mischievous when considered in reference to social progress; for only by such administrative work as brings the student into responsible relations with individuals, their circumstances, their powers of development, and their feelings is the judgment trained in what may be called the art of social life and administration.

The struggle between those who believed that the university should have nothing to do with the application of knowledge to realistic problems and those who saw the necessity for well-educated leaders who would have knowledge, ability to think, wisdom and judgment is clearly outlined here. To the Committee the only solution was to inaugurate a new and separate educational institution with a curriculum designed to use the best of university teaching combined with study in 'social obligation and administration'. In the light of that decision on the part of the Committee it is of interest to look at the proposed courses. The two-year comprehensive course was drawn up by Mr Urwick (later Professor Urwick) and was described as being of a standard suitable for students who could meet the intelligence of honour and better pass students at University. Its aim was to give an adequate basis of social theory, taking for granted that a good understanding of society was a necessary prerequisite for administrative work. It included lectures on various topics of 'social science and obligation', the development of society, social economics, some of the problems of social psychology and ethics, such as 'the formation of individual and social habit'. It included the history of the industrial classes and the history and methods of poor law relief and charity. The first year begins with 'principles directly bearing upon practice, concurrently with some practical work'. In connection with the practical work, further courses to supplement the lectures were to be given in the district offices and agencies bearing definitely on family and individual life, methods of assistance, and the general organization of aid and relief.

Mr Urwick's suggested course of lectures was divided into three general areas of knowledge which were to continue through the two years: (1) Principles directly bearing upon practice. (2) Theory of the Structure of Society. (3) Economic Principles.

Combined with these lectures and the reading outlined to go with them was the practical work. Miss Sewell proposed the following arrangements: (a) three months daily at a Charity Organisation Society office *under special guidance*. 'The Secretary to discuss certain definite economic and relief problems in connection with actual cases, and to organize expeditions to the various institutions used in relief work.' (b) a second term spent on Poor Law administration and observation of its working in one or more unions. (c) the remainder of year to be spent on local government and normal industrial and social conditions and institutions, together with some actual work under an experienced person in some form of charitable work not primarily relief work.

In connection with this plan, Mrs Bosanquet presented in some detail the practical work within a Charity Organisation Society office. Her outline follows closely the methods she presented in her earlier paper.[6] Students would be engaged in (1) Case-work, including study of case-papers, home visiting, inquiry work, interviewing applicants, preparation of treatment plans, etc. (2) District work – study of the community. (3) Organization, including organizing meetings, committees, lectures, inter-agency relationships, and certain social action activities, e.g. working on local government institutions, promoting the election of desirable candidates.

Mrs Bosanquet's plans resemble modern ideas of good

[6] See page 12.

general field work, including a training in skills and techniques, a knowledge of the community and its resources, and practice in administrative and organizational methods and implications.

Some criticism was raised within the Committee in reference to Mr Urwick's plan of lectures. The suggestion was made that they were not sufficiently sociological and further suggestions were made of books to supplement those already suggested. Also it was thought by some that the course should be more entirely related to conditions of industrial life and the growth of society and social duty. The Rev C. F. Rogers outlined such an alternative course. In the first year students were to have, first, the development of society, and the history of labour and outline of economic history. They were then to move on to present conditions of life and labour dealing first with the normal conditions of the industrial classes and secondly with the 'development of social duty' which would include poor law and charity history and general remedial measures. Mr Rogers thought the second year should be organized in detail around such topics as: (1) The family and organization – the family as the unit of social life and the relation of legal, charitable, and other agencies to it and each other. (2) The Child – legislation, agencies, problems. (3) The Adult – destitution, vagrancy, lunacy, handicaps of various kinds. (4) Women and the Aged – widows, rescue work, pensions, incurables. Mr Rogers also thought that special monographs should be written on many of these subjects and that the whole, of course, would be combined with the practical work as outlined by Miss Sewell and Mrs Bosanquet.

One cannot fail to recognize that Mr Rogers' plan comes the closest to outlining a professional course of study with the main emphasis placed on the problems and the remedies to be applied by those who know how to use them.

In addition to a two-year comprehensive course of study, the Committee also submitted in their report a short six-month course outlined by Miss Sewell and intended for large groups of charitable workers not really equipped by inclination, interest, or resources to do the longer course of study. This short course, more like an in-service training, was set up to give some lectures on relief and relief giving, elementary economics, history and administration of the Poor Law, and local government combined with a proportionately large amount of practical work. Other suggestions for this type of student included centreing the training in a Charity Organisation Society office and supplementing it with a simple course of practical lectures. Another short course of six lectures was outlined for men who were about to enter the Ministry and included the following subjects: The Family and the Standard of Life, Scope of Economics, Wants, Wages, Poor Law Relief and Destitution, Charity and Remedial Help. A further general programme of training for poor law officers was outlined by Mr W. Vallance, clerk to the Whitechapel Board of Guardians, and the Committee suggested that a small committee under the chairmanship of Mr Vallance be set up to study the matter further.

To implement all of these educational and training plans, the Committee recommended the appointment of a 'Director of Studies . . . to see and advise students and to arrange for their teaching'. They also recommended that the idea of establishing a 'trust' be abandoned in favour of a more flexible form of organization and suggested that the Social Education Committee should be registered under the Companies Act as a non-profit-making company and 'that the Association should be defined as an association for providing lectures and teaching; for promoting a knowledge of social science and economics, with special reference to social obligation and administration, issuing publications, providing scholarships, and contributing towards special investigations authorized, and to incur expenditure for all these and such other purposes as are consistent with its objects. . . .' Various other details of organization and finance were outlined and recommended, including a General Committee with an executive committee of 12, of whom two-thirds should be members of the Charity Organisation Society.

Events moved rapidly following this report. The following month the Council of the Charity Organisation Society entertained and passed a motion proposed by Thomas Mackay that the Special Committee on Social Education be a separate and independent Committee.[1] From that date our information becomes sketchy. Unfortunately the records of the Separate Committee and the School of Sociology and Social Economics which it became have been lost or were destroyed. We do know from the report of the Special Committee for 1902 that Miss Sharpley, who had been the full-time lecturer and tutor since the beginning of the Joint Committee in 1896, resigned in the Autumn of 1902 to become sub-warden of the Women's University Settlement and no replacement was made during the year because of the proposed re-organization. It should be noted that Mrs G. F. Hill was Honorary Secretary of the Joint Lectures Committee through all the years from 1896 and continued as Secretary when the new School of Sociology was established. She seems to have devoted an immense amount of time and work to the cause of training social workers.

Thus ended an era and thus was prepared with much promise a new age of professional education for social work. Originating in an effort to supply trained workers for various agencies working directly with people, the Joint Committee and the Special Committee of the Charity Organisation Society were led along by experience and conviction to the realization that something more was needed – education in broader fields of knowledge combined with practical application was the answer they found and which is professional education in contrast to merely technical

[1] *Minutes of the Council*, Charity Organisation Society, July 20, 1903.

training. That they failed to solve the problem of how to relate this new idea of education for modern social responsibilities to the older teaching within the Universities is understandable and not surprising in that the problem still remains unsolved in Britain. Probably it has been difficult to solve because of some confusion in not seeing clearly that there is a distinct difference between academic instruction in the social sciences and the professional application of knowledge gained in those fields. The Universities, even if they too are not clear in their thinking, are right in objecting to the mixing together of the academic and the professional. A knowledge of economics and social structure and political science are a necessary base of knowledge for the social worker. They should be studied as a scientific background just as the prospective physician learns physiology and anatomy. But this knowledge is not that which is applied in practical work to social problems any more than anatomy as such is used by the physician in his clinical work. Certain methods and skills must be taught upon this base of scientific knowledge which can be applied to help the individual meet his problems. Professional education must have three parts: (1) Academic education – in science and in philosophy which serve as a background and give the student a base of broad understanding; (2) Methods and skills, and (3) Applied practice and clinical work. An attempt to make the background content that which is applied practically merely confuses the issue.

That the Special Committee of the Charity Organisation Society were aware of this to some degree is evidenced in their proposed courses because these plans include all three elements of professional education. The main difficulty lay in the fact that skills and methods had not been well formulated as yet and, naturally, were not recognized as being something which could be taught in the classroom rather than gained through hit and miss experience in the field. This is particularly true of case work methods, but skills in administration and organization were recognized and planned for in the course of instruction. Close attention to Mrs Bosanquet's suggestions on practical work and the implementing of the Rev C. F. Rogers's idea of writing special monographs on problems and remedial measures probably would have led to a formulation of professional method.

CHAPTER III

THE SCHOOL OF SOCIOLOGY

As was pointed out above, the records of the School of Sociology are not available so that whatever information can be gleaned from various reports and papers must be used. The Annual Report of the Charity Organisation Society for 1903-04[1] indicates that the School was established to begin operations in the autumn of 1903. Mr E. J. Urwick was appointed Lecturer and Tutor. Courses of instruction in different branches of social economy had been arranged and classes had been organized with practical work in connection with a number of District Committees of the Charity Organisation Society. 'The formation of the School of Sociology has been a definite attempt to induce people *to think*, and not to shrink from applying theory to practical work.'

The 'introductory' lecture delivered by Mr Urwick in October, 1903 on 'Social Education of Yesterday and Today'[2] gives some indication of the thinking, aims and objectives and a considerable idea of the direction in which the development of training would proceed. He quotes Socrates in an opening statement: 'I think you will find that in all matters those who have the best repute, and are most looked up to, are amongst those who understand best; while the uninstructed have a bad name and are despised.' Mr

[1] *Thirty-fifth Annual Report of the Charity Organisation Society,* March 21, 1904.
[2] Reprinted in *Charity Organisation Review,* No. 83, November, 1903.

Urwick in following that thought impressed upon his audience the necessity for practitioners in any field to be well instructed: '. . . his methods must be made scientific, his practice must be founded upon a true knowledge of principles and law; and he – the practitioner – must himself acquire that knowledge and be trained in these methods.' He states that social workers are practitioners like physicians and surgeons and teachers, but that 'we are still in the rule-of-thumb stage, like the barber-surgeons of old, following customary methods, often without knowing whether they are good or bad'. Training in the past had amounted to little more than 'picking up fragments of experience under the guidance of other practitioners who have worked long enough to learn that some methods succeed while others fail'. He stated that this apprenticeship type of training had answered the needs of the time, but that new needs and changes were demanding something more comprehensive. Just as the emphasis in the Eighteenth Century was on freedom, in the Nineteenth Century on power and strength, so in our own time, the emphasis is on greater fulness of life, 'for a completer realization of the possibilities of social life'. Mr Urwick adds that 'there is a new knowledge; in it may be found the scientific basis for the social education we need; and it is essential that the worker should learn it'. Economics appeared as a science at the time of the industrial revolution, psychology arrived on the scene in time to be essential to the development of education and now sociology had its place to show the way for new social interests and 'as the interpreter of the complex social life which now for the first time has become an almost universal object of thought'. He divided the new knowledge into four parts: (1) The *natural history of society*. (2) That which dealt with how society and the individual grow and change and what they can and ought to grow and change into, or *social philosophy*. (3) The framework of economic necessities, or *social economics* and (4) knowledge of the mental processes on which development depends or *individual and social psychology*.

And in this statement Mr Urwick gives the general outlines of the scientific basis upon which the education of the social worker depended. Social workers, as he said, cannot be 'mere practitioners, leaving to others the task of understanding the theory on which their work is based'. He summarized in his final monumental paragraph as follows: 'He (the social worker) must learn to realize the slow growth that lies behind each present condition and fact; to see in the social structure, whole or part, of state or of institution, the expression of a vital meaning; to feel beneath the seemingly plastic relationships of social life the framework of economic necessities; and to find in each casual tendency and habit the effect of slowly changing mental processes. Not the training of the man of science, but the scientific attitude must be his; that at least is necessary if experience is to be used aright. And is it unreasonable to believe that experience so guided will lead to a higher level of administration, a surer touch in dealing with what we call our "social problems"; above all a better conception and fulfilment of our recognized social duties?'

A paper by Mr C. S. Loch, written in 1907,[2] includes a considerable amount of material from the reports of the School of Sociology and Economics for the years 1904-05 and 1905-06. He reviews the early teaching in social economics begun by the Women's University Settlement, which developed into the School of Sociology. He throws some interesting light on attitudes in various groups towards social problems in stating: 'The greater people were for large schemes and ignored "cases" — and have gone on doing so, I think. The lesser people seemed haunted with the idea that the poor were to be always with us, and that the individual poor were to be dealt with very much as each thought best. There was no conception that society had

[2] *Charity Organisation Society Pamphlets, 1898-1907.*

grown up like other things that come within the compass of our thought, and that in some way it was the expression of laws that we should have to understand and follow if a better state of things were to be the outcome of our action. . . .' The treatment of the individual medically was, at least so far as the hospital was concerned, a more or less scientific matter; but the treatment of the individual socially was not a scientific matter. Nor was there, I think, any general conception that new statutes, if they were to have a good effect, could only be grounded on a wide knowledge of individuals and their lives and possibilities.'

In the light of the fifty years' experience following these statements, it can be said that Mr Urwick's outline of the basic knowledge necessary for social workers, together with Mr Loch's statement of the need for scientific method in the social treatment of the individual constitute a sound professional education plan for social workers.

We are indebted to Mr Loch's paper for certain facts and statistics about the School of Sociology in its beginning years. In 1904-05 there were sixteen students, ten of whom were 'full-time'; and in 1905-06 there were twenty-one, of whom sixteen completed a full course. Dr James Bonar gave the inaugural address in 1904-05. The Michaelmas Term lectures included: 'London and Londoners' and 'Theories and Methods of Social Improvement' by Mr Urwick; 'Poor Relief in Relation to Recent History and Present Conditions in France and England'; 'Some Economic Questions' by Miss E. A. Pearson, of Lady Margaret Hall Settlement; and 'Social Legislation' by Miss Margaret Sewell.

The Session of 1905-06 was opened by an inaugural address by M. Edmond Demolins. Other lectures were given as follows: 'Good Citizenship', by the Bishop of Stepney and others; 'The Improvement of the Conditions of the Poor', by Mr A. H. Paterson; 'Friendly Societies and Other Methods of Thrift', by Mr Edward Brabrook, C.B.; 'Social and Industrial Difficulties of the Present Day'; 'An Introductory Course in the Divisions of Sociological Study and Literature'; 'Individualism and Socialism, Economic and Political'; a 'Discussion Class', by Mr Urwick; 'The Principles Underlying Social Work', by Mrs Frank Ogilvey; and an introductory course for those interested mainly in practical work, by Miss Plater.

Mr Loch points out that the work of the School was divided into three departments: (1) Social Theory and Administration, including history and theory of social and industrial movements, reforms, economic theory, industrial history, outlines of political science, and administration of charity and poor law. (2) Sociology, including analysis of social structures, history and theory of social growth and change, theory of social forces, and (3) Specialized department of practical instruction in poor law administration under a separate committee of the School. Each department was intended for a separate class of students. The first for those primarily interested in social betterment, the second for a smaller group of more systematic students, and the third for poor law officers and those wishing to enter that field.

The practical work was arranged in various societies and agencies with most of the students spending a few months in a Charity Organisation Society office. This is in line with our present-day thinking that the first field work training of students is best given in general family work.

Some lectures and classes in the School were open to the public, but classes, in contrast to lectures, were limited to twenty students. Mr Loch makes an observation about qualification of staff: 'The lectures should be given by men and women who have by their knowledge of affairs and experience, as well as by their general intellectual ability, proved their right to be teachers in this branch of science. The teachers should themselves have passed through the severe discipline of case work; for in my opinion there is no discipline like that, either for the teacher or the pupil.

Whatever originality of treatment the future may bring forth is not likely, I think, to come from generalities of passing opinion, but from actual observation and experiment in regard to individual cases and in regard to groups of individuals.' In the years following, there has been an increasing emphasis on the necessity for the teachers of professional content to be themselves qualified social workers.

That the founders of the School of Sociology had broader ideas than the mere training of social workers and saw the need for the dissemination of social knowledge to the general public, is evidenced from time to time in the writings of C. S. Loch, but also particularly in the 1904 inaugural address of Dr James Bonar,[4] and in a paper read to the School by Mr John N. Muirhead, of Birmingham, on December 5, 1904.[5] Dr Bonar touched on, and Mr Muirhead expanded, the idea of the necessity for reaching both the population generally and the teachers in elementary and secondary schools so that young people would be recruited at an early age to the ranks of those who were concerned and interested in social questions and methods of attacking social problems. In the same fashion, perhaps, as the medical profession has concerned itself with seeing that knowledge and understanding of health and illness be given to ordinary lay people, so these pioneers in the social field recognized the essentially professional requirement of making generally available knowledge and understanding in their field. Although professional practitioners in any field must, because of their technical skills, be a class apart, they cannot exist nor practise their skills unless the people generally have an understanding of the problems and the necessity

[4] Published in the *Charity Organisation Review*, No. 95, November, 1904.
[5] Published in the *Charity Organisation Review*, No. 98, February, 1905.

for the expert technique as well as an appreciation of and respect for the results of practice.

We must assume that the School of Sociology continued to develop until 1912 along the lines laid down in these earlier years. In fact various brief notes in the Charity Organisation Review from year to year indicate that such was the case. The education offered in the School through lectures, classes and practical work was held out as the basic general training of social workers and was not confused with special vocational training for a specific job. It will be remembered that the training offered for Poor Law officers, which was of the latter category, was kept separate and under the direction of a special committee of the School. The Charity Organisation Society, and, we can assume, other agencies, like the Settlements, accepted this premise and arranged for specific training on the job (it would be called orientation or in-service training today) for all new graduates who joined the staff. Those who became staff members of the Charity Organisation Society without preparation were given the opportunity of attending lectures of the School of Sociology, and we learn from the Forty-first Annual Report of the Society[6] that the School was beginning to arrange for local extension centres for lectures and teaching. The Charity Organisation Society itself conducted many discussion groups and 'reading circles' as a part of its in-service training. Thus by 1910 at least, and probably much earlier, it was clear that several levels and kinds of education and training for social work were necessary: full-time professional education, part-time study extension classes, orientation and in-service training.[7]

The Session of 1911-12 marks the last year of independent

[6] *Forty-first Annual Report of the Charity Organisation Society*, April 25, 1910.
[7] See: E. L. Younghusband. *Social Work in Britain*, Chapter XIII (Carnegie United Kingdom Trust, 1951), for a statement of the need for such a variety of preparations in social work at the present time.

existence of the School of Sociology. The inaugural address was given by Dr Bernard Bosanquet, and a brief note in the Charity Organisation Review[8] indicates that preliminary lectures were to be given by Professor Urwick; a course in 'Recent Social Legislation' by Mr R. C. Davison; three historical courses by Professor Urwick; and 'Social Ethics and Philosophy' by Miss Pearson.

It is not clear how the School was financed, although from the original plans in the Special Committee's report in 1903 it was recommended that 'efforts would be made to raise a fund producing at least £300 a year, and, in addition, annual voluntary contributions would be raised'. Mention of fees paid by students was made at various times. That the School suffered from financial difficulties is evidenced by a special grant of £50 made to it by the Charity Organisation Society in 1906.[9]

[8] *Charity Organisation Review*, October, 1911.
[9] *Minutes of the Council*, Charity Organisation Society, July 30, 1906.

CHAPTER IV

THE AMALGAMATION

ALTHOUGH the available records do not clearly indicate what were the immediate precipitating factors in bringing about the amalgamation of the School of Sociology with the London School of Economics, it is stated and implied that finance had much to do with the move. The Minutes of the Council[1] included a statement on the matter as a point of information. Mr B. Bosanquet, Chairman of the School, gave the Council an explanation of the reasons for the move. The Minutes state: 'He thought that the work which had been done by the School of Sociology had been very good in all its branches, but the rooms and the financial sources were quite inadequate. He had always regarded the practical work in connection with the School as being the great thing, and this work would be continued on the same lines by the London School of Economics.' The subject is closed with the remark by Lord Sanderson in which he said he hoped that the 'attention of the London School of Economics would be drawn to the fact that the Society possessed a library dealing with social questions'.

The Annual Report of the Society also makes note of the change.[2] It states that new arrangements had been made for carrying on the School. Professor Urwick had been its

[1] *Minutes of the Council,* Charity Organisation Society, July 22, 1912.
[2] *Forty-fourth Annual Report of the Charity Organisation Society,* June 2, 1913.

Director since the beginning and Mrs G. F. Hill its Hon. Secretary. 'The policy of the School . . . has been to combine courses of practical instruction at District Committees of the Society with courses of lectures. In this joint education of practice and teaching, which is now adopted at other schools, the School of Sociology has led the way.' Mention is made of the fact that the London School of Economics had made the proposal to take over the School of Sociology and form out of it a Department of Social Science and Administration. The School of Sociology as an entirely voluntary institution was unable to raise the funds to continue and expand its work, and it was conceded that the School of Economics had ample funds for the purpose. In the arrangements made, it was agreed that the new department would be under the direction of Professor Urwick, and that for two years the staff and the general arrangements would remain as they had been. The report adds that the success of the department would depend 'on its Director having been himself trained in the practical duties of case work and co-operation. Thus trained he acquires a careful administrative judgment, which may check and supplement the teaching of the social sciences'. The writer of the report highly recommends Professor Urwick in this respect. 'By a strange perversity as it seems, however, sociologists and economists are frequently led to deal with questions of social science without acquiring at first hand any careful and consistent knowledge of the facts and conditions of personal and social life in the daily competition and struggle of the common people, the poor, the very poor, who form the largest part of the population.' The course of training for Poor Law officers which had been conducted by the School of Sociology was to be carried on independently by a joint committee of the National Poor Law Officers Association and of the late School.

The School of Sociology in making the arrangements to have the staff and general plan of education continued for a period of two years obviously was hoping to protect the professional quality of the scheme from being swallowed up by theoretical economics and sociology. It is apparent that there was a realization that two completely different approaches existed – one that of academic teaching and a second which was professional, but the real difference between the two was not yet clearly defined. The only distinction expressed seems to be that of practicality, or an application of economic and social principles in contrast to purely theoretical study. Actual methods and skills of helping people as individuals or as groups, which is, after all, the core of professional education, were not recognized as the distinguishing feature, but were considered as a more or less incidental part of the 'practical work'. Why this was so can be easily seen if one looks at the development of the case work method in the history of the Charity Organisation Society. The Society made no pretence of being primarily concerned with case work until World War I.[8] Its paid or professional staff were district secretaries who were organizers not case workers. Any case work, although the importance of it was not underestimated, was left entirely to volunteers, friendly visitors and district church visitors. Although it was recognized that friendly visitors had to be 'trained', one could hardly expect that a teachable system of professional method would be developed through the practice of volunteers. Why methods of organization and administration did not become the professional core of studies is a little more difficult to understand because they could have served the same purpose in the development of professional education. With the transfer of what had begun as a professional educational plan for social workers to an academic institution without a clear understanding

[8] See: *Fifty-first Annual Report of the Charity Organisation Society*, in which case work is first recognized as a function of the Charity Organisation Society.

of the differences involved, only one result could obtain: The professional aspects would become less important and the academic and theoretical more important.

The London School of Economics, however, long before the amalgamation had advertised its lectures in Sociology as of interest to social workers, listing poor law guardians, committee members of philanthropic societies, district visitors among others who might be interested.[4] It is interesting to note also that certain special lectures were introduced from time to time. Professor Urwick in 1905-06 gave a series on 'Economic Basis of Social Relations'. Mr Webb lectured on Poor Law History; and Mr and Mrs Webb alternately gave lectures in 'Methods of Social Investigation' from 1905-06 to 1910-11.

The Calendar of the London School of Economics for 1912-13 makes a statement regarding the amalgamation and indicates the policy which would be pursued:

'The provision of additional accommodation was rendered essential by the creation of a new department, that of Social Science and Administration, in the work of the School. This department will continue the work carried on for nine years by the School of Sociology and Social Economics which merged in the School of Economics and Political Science in the end of July 1912.'[5]

The Calendar continues: 'This department is intended for those who wish to prepare themselves to engage in the many forms of social and charitable effort. Its methods will follow those which have been in use for nine years at the School of Sociology. . . . A large proportion of the training will consist in giving the students first-hand experience of social work. This experience will be afforded by association with Children's Care Committee, Skilled Employment Associations, Labour Exchanges, Committees of the Charity

[4] *Calendar*, London School of Economics, 1904-05.
[5] *Calendar*, London School of Economics, 1912-13, p. 36.

Organisation Society, Rent Collecting, Provident Visiting, Club Management, special inquiries into industrial conditions and various branches of settlement work – the student always being under the guidance of experienced social workers. The experience thus gained will form a part of a scheme of education by lectures, class teaching and individual tuition at the London School of Economics.'

The Calendar further emphasizes that the academic teaching was to be 'intimately connected' with the lessons learned by the student in his practical work. Of particular note is the provision for individual tuition: 'The students are placed under the charge of a tutor, who will advise them as to the best forms of practical work, and ensure that this work is made of educational value.'[6] From this statement one would gather that the tutors were to be primarily concerned with the practical work and the integration of it with the academic studies. There is no indication in the later history of the Department that this idea was carried out; nor that any arrangement was ever made for the tutors to move out into the field in order to actually instruct in practical work, thus ensuring the educational value of that part of the plan.

For two years, as was agreed, the scheme for the education of social workers was continued as the School of Sociology had arranged it. In addition to regular courses in economics, sociology, politics, statistics and law there were special lectures in the department which might very well be designated as social work or professional courses: Introduction to Social Work and Study: Types of State Assistance; Social Movements of Recent Times; and Working Class Life. This was a one-year course with arrangements possible for students who wished to continue for a second year.

In these earliest years of the Social Science Department, the Calendar makes clear that the course is divided equally

---

[6] *Calendar*, London School of Economics, 1912-13, p. 81.

between practical and academic work, and this statement is repeated during the years that Professor Urwick remained in charge. It is not within the purposes of this paper to write the history of the Social Science Department of the London School of Economics, but rather its antecedents, and to draw upon some parts of its history as a matter of comparison. In 1917-18 the Department became the Ratan Tata Department of Social Science and Administration in that the Ratan Tata Foundation assumed the complete financing. Previously the Foundation had made available certain lectures and research facilities for advanced students in the Department. A glance at the lectures and classes required for the Certificate in 1917-18[1] will show that the emphasis upon professional and practical application was present and developing.

The curriculum can be divided into three sections. The first grouping of courses is intended to give a background knowledge in the social sciences, including: Economic History, Social History from 1760, Social Philosophy, Application of Economic Principles to Social Questions, Social Economics, Comparative and Social Psychology. A second group can be seen to include social problems and the organization of the social services: Social and Industrial Problems, Social Institutions, Care Committee Work under the Education Authority, New Forms of Social Effort, the Conditions upon which the maintenance of Health in Factory and Home Depends. The third section includes courses clearly designed as methods in case work, administration, and community work: Preparatory Class in Case Work and Methods of Charitable Administration; Special Tutorial Class (short lectures, talks and discussion once a week for the entire session); Introductory Course on Practical Work and Observation and the Social and Industrial Characteristics of London; a Historical and Critical Account of Some

[1] *Calendar*, London School of Economics, 1917-18.

Principles of Social Management; Elementary Statistical Methods.

However, almost immediately after the amalgamation of the School of Sociology with the School of Economics, the Charity Organisation Society felt the necessity of increasing its own training plans. That the Social Science Department of the School of Economics did not meet the need for training the practitioner is evidenced by the numbers of other agencies and institutions which co-operated with the Charity Organisation Society during this period in a variety of training schemes. By 1915, under pressure from various groups. the Charity Organisation Society had organized a formal, twelve-month training course. A certificate was to be granted for the successful completion of it. That the Charity Organisation Society was still campaigning for professional education, including a high level of practical clinical work, is evidenced in the following statement from the Forty-seventh Annual Report (1914-15):

'With so much give and take and mutual appreciation in so large a group of extensive agencies, it seems not too much to hope that the bodies doing practical social work may be able to evolve among them one or more authorities in such combined strength as to assure recognition. Should London University reach the point of offering a degree in Competence for Social Service, this federation of social agencies interested in training should be able to negotiate on equal terms with the teachers of theory. It should be possible to make similar arrangements with Oxford and Cambridge to those by which men taking the M.D. degrees of those Universities get their practical training in London hospitals.'[8]

A training Committee was organized and lectures and practical work were arranged. An honorary tutor, Miss Edith Pearson, was placed in charge of the students. One would

[8] *Forty-seventh Annual Report of the Charity Organisation Society*, April 10, 1916.

almost think one was reading about the earlier period before 1903 if the date of the report were not carefully noted. The Committee announced that they wanted it 'understood that these lectures form no part of a plan to revive the School of Sociology. They are an attempt to supplement such explanations of the aims and conditions of their case work as the secretaries would give in the offices if time permitted.'

The first group of six students to complete the new training course were granted their certificates in the summer of 1916. In that year, too, arrangements were made for a co-operative scheme with Bedford College. The Forty-eighth Annual Report explains: 'While appreciating the theoretical instruction given at the London School of Economics, and utilizing it for its students, the Committee were at a loss to find a course on some of the practical aspects of social work, and also to find theoretical courses for students beginning training after Christmas.'[9]

The following year it was reported that the joint Bedford College and Charity Organisation Society scheme was proving extremely popular with an average attendance of over a hundred.[10] With the success of the new certificate course in Charity Organisation Society training combined with lectures at Bedford College, the Society reassured itself again that the proper training for social work was a professional scheme of education involving both 'historical and academic explanation in the lecture rooms of a university' and practice work in the field under the guidance of experienced social workers. The necessity of a different and separate kind of institution for educating social workers was expressed (as it had been in 1903) in the 1919 report: 'No sounder contribution to reconstruction could be made than an endowment fund to enable suitable people to go

[9] *Forty-eighth Annual Report of the Charity Organisation Society*, March 7, 1917.
[10] *Forty-ninth Annual Report of the Charity Organisation Society*, March 18, 1918.

through a really adequate training for this great work."[11]

The movement begun in 1903 and brought to a culmination in 1912 to introduce social work training into the universities resulted in two things: An increasing emphasis through the years upon academic and theoretical education on the one hand, and new and greater numbers of training schemes outside the universities and within the agencies on the other.

That this line of development has continued is shown rather clearly by the training provided currently in the Social Science Department of the London School of Economics. A brief glance at the Calendar for 1951-52 shows that the old unresolved conflict between training for practice and general academic education is still present:

'The Certificate awarded to students in the Department of Social Science and Administration is meant primarily for men and women who wish to devote themselves professionally to work in connection with the statutory or voluntary social services, or in the personnel and welfare departments of industry. The course is designed to give at the same time a general education in the field of social science.'[12]

The four subjects required for examination: Social Economics, History, Social Philosophy and Psychology, and Social Administration[13] indicate a weighting in favour of social and economic theory and background, resulting probably in more nearly meeting the second objective: 'to give at the same time, a general education in the field of social science.' The picture of what is happening is clearer, too, when one notes that a special certificate is issued to students who complete a course for social workers in mental health, that there is a special child care course, and that there is a grouping of courses for personnel management

[11] *Fiftieth Annual Report of the Charity Organisation Society*, March 24, 1919.
[12] *Calendar*, London School of Economics, 1951-52, p. 140.
[13] Ibid, p. 141.

students. The tendency seems to be to make social science a general background of preparation for special courses concerned primarily with professional method and practice.

CHAPTER V

AFTERTHOUGHT

A SUMMARY of the entire story shows a recurring theme. The period before 1903, marked by original training schemes within the agencies, led naturally to a recognition for the need of broader preparation. The independent school established to meet that need had all the elements of professional education in its curriculum at its inception. Why it was not possible to secure adequate financial support for the School of Sociology is not clear. There is, however, a distinct connection between the fact that professional methods and skills were not developed and formulated for teaching within the School and the fact that the curricula gradually became more theoretical. This is inferred from the increased emphasis on training practitioners within the Charity Organisation Society even before the amalgamation. Immediately following that event, other agencies joined with the Charity Organisation Society and new training plans were put in motion resulting in the twelve-months' certificate course. And for a second time, training in professional methods was centred in the agencies. Within a few years, by 1919 that is, the need for an endowed school which would combine the broad academic teaching of the university with the training in method and practice was again expressed.

From that time a multitude of technical training schemes sponsored by government departments and voluntary agencies have sprung up to meet the need of the new social services for qualified practitioners. Once more such agency training plans have led, just as in the period before 1903 and before 1919, to a recognition of the need for a school to teach professional social work on a university level. The two reports[1] issued by the Carnegie United Kingdom Trust in 1947 and 1951, based upon careful studies of the problem, outline clearly the necessity of and plans for such a school.

In the movement before 1903 and in each succeeding period when the establishment of a school of social work has been urged, emphasis has been placed on the need for a broad university preparation combined with technical knowledge and practice. The importance of education in the social sciences for social workers has been recognized and has been established over the years. Without doubt, the more technical training offered under the auspices of agencies and departments has improved and advanced with each era. Confusion still exists as to just how the two can be brought logically together. This confusion arises mainly because the whole of professional content has not been recognized nor presented to the universities as professional education rather than vocational or technical training.

Professional education in any field includes: *first*, a base of scientific, theoretical and philosophical knowledge. For social work that means academic study in sociology, economics, anthropology, psychology, and political science; secondly, an application of these in terms of problems and remedies. In social work that would be the social problems of individuals and groups along with the institutions, organizations, and services set up to meet these problems; thirdly, methods and skills, and in social work these are: casework, group work, administration, research, and social action.

Some of this content should be acquired in ordinary university lectures as a background or pre-professional base.

[1] Eileen L. Younghusband, *Report on the Employment and Training of Social Workers*, 1947 (*Carnegie United Kingdom Trust*) and *Social Work in Britain*, 1951 (C.U.K.T.).

Some can be given only in a specially organized and integrated professional curriculum. Where the line is drawn between the two depends somewhat upon how far any particular university goes in teaching applied social sciences, or how much of the second division stated above (problems and remedies) is incorporated into the theoretical social science teaching. The third section of professional content can only be taught clinically, that is, through applied work under direction in the field and in discussion classes.

Technical or vocational training in social work consists of the third division with some of the second, resulting in persons who know mainly how to do certain things. There is always the danger of their developing rule-of-thumb methods and of not knowing why they do what they do, nor if what they do is right or wrong. Professional education must be squarely based upon a scientific and theoretical content. Both the broader base and the technical training have been developing soundly but separately over the years. The final step of bringing them together must be made if the recurring circles of the past are to be broken.

APPENDIX I

The Training of Volunteers[1]

By

Mrs DUNN GARDNER

BEFORE those in charge of the District Committees of the C.O.S. can be expected to devote themselves to the difficult and troublesome task of Training Volunteer Workers, they must be really convinced that this is one of their chief and most important duties.

We are very fond of reiterating that the C.O.S. is an organizing and not a relief Society, but in practice we of the District Committees feel very loth to undertake the constant daily trouble involved in bringing about this organization. We are willing enough to have a try to organize some large institution, or local charity, or parish meeting, or benevolent society – to organize, in fact, *en bloc* – but when it becomes a question of organizing individuals – that is to say, of convincing them, one by one, that our principles are true, and of inducing them to guide their actions by these principles, we are most of us inclined to shirk the task. I believe myself that the wholesale system of doing things is as false when applied to organization as when applied to relief, and that important bodies can only be truly won over to our side by

[1] Read to the Council of the Charity Organisation Society, November 26, 1894, and printed in the C.O.S. *Occasional Papers* – First Series – No. 46.

carefully and thoroughly dealing with the individuals who compose them.

We must at once dismiss from our minds the idea that workers are to be trained only with a view to their being useful to their trainers. Often when the subject of volunteers is being discussed I have heard people say, 'Oh, I would so much rather do the work myself.' Of course they would – it would take half the time, and less than half the trouble, of getting someone else to do it – but the result attained would be quite different. The district offices of the C.O.S. exist not to get their own special office work well done, nor to assist a certain number of cases every year, but to improve the general condition of the poor, in their own particular district, and throughout London. The Committee largely devote their energies to relief work because this is the chief means at their disposal for the organization of those individuals by whom it is hoped that the improvement may be brought about. One of the best methods of teaching is the giving of object lessons; and each case carefully and efficiently dealt with by a C.O.S. Committee ought to be an object lesson in the best methods of charity. Once let this principle be accepted, and we see our offices, instead of being Relief Societies working in rivalry with other Relief Societies, and competing with them for funds, for workers, and even for cases – instead of this, we see them become what I believe they were meant to be – and what they must be to achieve their object – Schools of True Charity. The Secretary at one of these schools, of course, will not expect a new pupil to relieve him of his work, but the advent of each learner will mean to him new duties and new responsibilities. He will cease to regard each pupil, who leaves after his course is over, as one on whom the labours of training have been wasted; for he will know that it is away from the old school, that the exercise of the principles taught there are most needed; and he will pride himself on the number of workers trained in the science of Charity, whom he can afford to send out as missionaries, while he still keeps his own establishment up to a high standard of efficiency.

Regarding C.O.S. offices from this point of view, the practical question presents itself, what is it best to do with new workers? And to answer this question, we must, I think, divide our new workers into two classes – those who offer their help to the C.O.S., and those who are already at work in the district. We will begin with the first class, who are far the easier to deal with, though much I say about them is applicable to the other class, too.

Now, I should like to lay special stress on two points. One is that the first thing to do with new workers is to *interest* them: if we fail to do this I think we shall not get far in training them. And the second point to which I want to draw attention goes hand in hand with the first, and it is that you must make all workers – old as well as new, for the matter of that – feel their own *Responsibility*. It is useless to expect anyone to go on regularly doing anything unless he feels that it makes some difference to somebody whether he does it or not. No doubt his attendance must often involve considerable personal inconvenience, and, if he finds that things go on equally well, whether he does or does not keep his engagements, it is only natural that he should stay away when it is difficult for him to come – but once let him be sure that inconvenience, or delay, or suffering, will follow on his failing to do what he has undertaken, and you will find he is very unlikely to let anything stand in the way of his work.

Bearing then in mind these two points, that men and women if they are to stick to voluntary work must be interested in it, and must recognize their own share of responsibility in what is being done, we will go on to deal with our new worker.

The Secretary has generally from the very first two courses open to him. Probably there is some bit of work at the office which is standing over till it can get taken in hand. The new worker may have this bit of work explained to him, and may be set down to carry it on. If he happens to take to it, well and good; if not, why then he will soon leave off coming to the office, and the same bit of work will be ready to hand to choke off the next energetic aspirant after employment (I can recommend the loan books as a very valuable extinguisher of enthusiasm – copying numerous begging letters, on an old case long since closed except from a money point of view, is also not bad). Or, instead of instructing him in this special bit of work, the Secretary may, to the best of his ability, try to train the newcomer, not for any special work, but for work itself; may, in fact, teach him not to make the head of the pin, or the point of the pin, but the whole article. To do this it is desirable that all new workers should go through the whole routine of the office, should open letters and answer them, should find case papers, and write them up, should deal with applicants, take loan money, enter up the different books, and see that inquiries from other Committees have been properly dealt with – indeed, I would like everyone who comes to work at a C.O.S. office to learn as far as possible the duties of a Secretary, so as to be able if required to carry on any of them. One great gain of this system is that it does away with the notion which sometimes prevails, that there is something sacred about case papers and office documents, and that they should never be interfered with except under the special directions of the Secretary or Agent. If every worker has free access to papers, it will soon be understood that they exist not for the special information of the Secretary, but for the use of the whole Committee, and that they must be so kept as to be intelligible to all.

Of course, all this involves a great deal of inspection, and calls for constant patience and tact on the part of the Secretary (for instance, he will often find the letter about the Notice B Committee case, of the boy Jones, carefully put away in the Pension box, on the case of widow Jones), but ill results from such mistakes are easily guarded against by proper supervision. In letter-writing it may be a long time before any letter written by a newcomer can be sent out, and often the Secretary will have to spend part of his afternoon in re-writing the letters produced by volunteers in the morning. But this only lasts for a time, a time varying in length with each worker; for let us always remember that our workers have quite as varied natures as our applicants, and require to be dealt with in quite as varied a manner. Sometimes a new worker becomes useful in the office within a week of his coming; sometimes it is a month, or even a year, before any work he does has any practical value in really helping on the business of the Committee. Everyone before deciding on his future work should, I think, do a certain amount of visiting, and the best way I know of arranging for this is to get one of the most experienced S.R.D. almoners to take the new worker on her rounds a few times. More practical knowledge can be gained during one morning passed in the homes of the poor with a trained visitor, than in listening at the office to any amount of precepts about visiting. When the new worker has seen something of all that is being done at a C.O.S. office, he is in a position to decide for what branch of the work he feels most interest and is most suited.

For the full utilization and training of volunteers, I think it is a good plan to divide up the work of a Charity Organisation Society office as much as possible, placing each department under the special care of some one member of Committee who is responsible for its good working to the Secretary, who in his turn is responsible to the Committee. I would suggest that such departments may be formed:

For all matters connected with finance
For pension
For children boarded-out and in homes

For surgical cases

For convalescent cases

For loan cases

For invalid children

For cases arising in connection with the School Board. No office would, I think, need all these departments; they are only meant as suggestions.

Every member in charge of such department, and every visitor or almoner in charge of a special parish, should be encouraged to have an understudy for his part. By this I mean that he should have some other worker in training, under him, who will help in the special work, and will be able, in the event of the head of the department being called away, to step into his place. Head workers should often consider what would happen to their special branch of our business should they have to be absent for several months; and the Secretary will do well, I think, to caution them against making themselves indispensable.

This dividing up of the office work, besides giving a large field for the responsible employment of volunteers, relieves the Secretary of much routine work, and so sets free his time for the training of new workers. It is quite wrong, I think, to expect that the Secretary of any Committee should do the bulk of the casework. Though he must be cognisant of all that goes on in the office, he should himself, I think, only carry on just enough of it to keep the work up to that high standard of efficiency on which he must depend for an illustration of the truth of those principles which have called the Charity Organisation Society into existence.

Now we will pass on to the other class of workers we have to deal with at our C.O.S. offices – those already at work in the district. These are very difficult to get into touch with at all, but we cannot lay too much stress on the importance of organizing their efforts. They are chiefly, I think, City missionaries, district visitors, and ladies connected with the I.C.A.A., the M.A.B.Y.S., and with Evening Clubs. The time they wish to devote to charitable work is already occupied, they have their distinct interests, and they only come into our office by chance, probably over some case in which they are interested. I have found that the first thing to do with a local worker is to dispel the idea that the C.O.S. regards him as an intruder. He will apologize over and over again for taking up the Secretary's time, and will be profuse in his thanks if some slight trouble is taken for him. I have often found it almost impossible to get him to realize that the chief object of the existence of a C.O.S. office is to afford information, and to give advice, and to endeavour to strengthen the efforts already being made for good, and that, far from wishing to supersede local effort, our chief desire is to strengthen it.

If a case brought by a local worker proves helpable, it is very desirable to get the worker to carry on the case for the Committee, to explain to him that the opinion of one who has known the case for a long while will be much valued by the Committee, and that the fact that he is willing to continue indefinitely visiting the case will have considerable weight in the Committee's decision. When the case is a well-known one, which has been refused over and over again as unhelpable, there is nothing to do, I think, but to go through the old papers carefully and thoroughly with the local worker, trying to make clear why the case could not be helped, and to explain that if, now, any fresh facts can be brought to light to prove the past decision was wrong, the Committee are quite willing to go afresh into the matter.

When a local worker does come to the office it is desirable to take the opportunity of talking over with him any other cases in which he is at all likely to be interested, and if possible to get him to do something for the Committee, on any one of them, e.g. to collect a loan, or take a pension, or instil temperance. Very often a local worker is glad of some special information about benefit clubs, or evening classes, or the M.A.B.Y.S. offices, or hospitals. Some of them, especially District Visitors, often seem wonderfully ignorant of the district in which they are working. They are glad, too, sometimes of some C.O.S. papers, such as that on the 'Three Clubs'. After a few calls, the local worker may be induced to come to Committee to hear his own case discussed, and will perhaps stay on to listen to those of others living in the parish in which he is interested. I do not myself think it is much good to get quite new workers to attend long Committee meetings. The quick succession of long cases, presented in an unknown form, conveys very little at first. (I remember a lady telling me that the idea she carried away from the first C.O.S. Committee meeting she ever attended, was what a wonderful man R.O. must be. He seemed to be expected to know something of every family, and was helping or had helped so many.) When new workers do begin to attend Committee meetings, I think they should always sit where they can look over the case papers, and if they will, it is a good plan to get them to write the decisions. Every case which a local worker can be induced to carry through for the Committee is a great deal gained. Nothing is so likely to make him dissatisfied with incomplete trifling as to take part in thoroughly good work. Efforts should be made to let him see practically the better results of thorough work.

Don't let it be thought for a moment that I mean these remarks to apply to all local workers. There are men and women in some districts who are engaged in improving the condition of the poor, quite as thoroughly and as efficiently as we are, and who often, I am afraid, regard us with some suspicion. When they can be induced to come to us, with their wide local knowledge, their long experience gained by daily life amongst the poor, and their different standpoint from ours, they may have to learn from us a little about our special forms and formalities, but in wider matters it is they who will have to teach. As long as such men are at work, and hold aloof from us, we must feel that we have somehow failed to find quite the right way to organize charity.

I have not spoken of the importance of reading in the training of all workers. Every C.O.S. office, I suppose, has a few books it lends to its new recruits. I should like to see these few books become a real library in every case; and if there were a proper supply of books there would be no difficulty, I think, in getting them read. It is, however, practically no easy matter to procure new books for the office. If we buy them our General Fund has to pay, and our balance sheet will look all the worse for it next year. It would be nice to suggest to our next would-be benefactor that he should present the Society with thirty-nine suitable little libraries.

I have spoken throughout as though the training of workers depended entirely on the Secretary; let me therefore explain that I regard the Secretary only as the person who carried out the wishes of his Committee, and that in this, as in all else, a Secretary acting without the hearty co-operation of his Committeee is in a great measure powerless for good.

In conclusion, I should like again to point out that for the improvement of the general condition of the poor we do not want to produce only enough trained workers to carry on our own office work, but to make all work in our different districts efficient. Trained workers are needed to serve as Guardians; to visit the workhouse and infirmary; to act as school managers and members of Notice B Committees; to take part in the management of School Banks and Collecting Banks; to visit in connection with the I.C.A.A., the M.A.B.Y.S. and the G.F.S., and with the many Reformatory and Rescue Societies; to work under the clergy and ministers; to act as visitors to the hospitals, and as workers for the C.C.H.F., for Evening Clubs for boys and girls, for Sanitary Aid Committees, and for many other purposes. Those in charge of our District Offices have under their control the means of training these workers. They will know whether they have hitherto made the most of the trust confided to them.

Extracts from the

FIRST REPORT OF THE COMMITTEE ON TRAINING[1]

adopted by the Council of the Charity Organisation Society,
December 12, 1898

THIS Committee was appointed on the 28th day of June,
1897. It has met eleven times, and has held a Conference of
some of the most experienced members of District Committees, at which the subject of training in its various
aspects was fully discussed. It has already made a recom-
mendation to the Administrative Committee with regard to
a proposed course of instruction for district and honorary
secretaries, which has been adopted by the Administrative
Committee. It now begs to present an introductory report
and some recommendations.

It is possibly only of late years that the importance of
'training' as a special feature of charity organization has
been at all generally recognized. Formerly probably it was
considered that the work itself would be sufficiently educational, and that charity organizers would be produced auto-
matically. Time, however, and experience, and the comparison of the educational results of the work of one Committee with those of another, have abundantly shown that
where insufficient attention is given to the matter there is
apt to be great waste of power and eventual loss to the
Society.

It is hardly necessary to dwell upon the importance of the
question. It is self-evident that unless the forces at the dis-

[1] Printed in *C.O.S. Occasional Papers* – Second Series, Paper No. 11.

posal of the Society are made thoroughly efficient they can never exercise any adequate influence upon outside opinion – unless the tree is sound at heart it will never throw out vigorous branches. It has been said more than once that training and charity organization are one and the same. There can be no doubt that every trained charity organizer becomes in his turn a centre of charity organization effective in proportion to his grasp of principle and strength of conviction.

The word 'training' may be interpreted to cover the whole field of proselytization amongst those who attend District Committees, and to include the training of clergy, district visitors, and outside workers of every sort; or it may be held to apply primarily to the education and instruction of executive members of the Society. The importance of training outside workers cannot, of course, be exaggerated, but for the purposes of this report the training of executive members of the Society must be the chief consideration.

The training of both classes of workers is, of course, intimately connected and is, up to a certain point, identical. That of executive members, however, includes many practical details and technicalities which do not come within the scope of outside workers, and it includes the acceptance of a larger measure of personal responsibility. It is, moreover, to executive members that we must look in the long run to influence and educate those whose work amongst the poor lies in other directions.

The appointment of the Committee was due to the belief that the training of executive members of the Society had not hitherto been so complete as it might be, and that the ventilation of the subject would lead to a higher standard of efficiency. The general impression derived from the discussion at the Conference already alluded to was that there still prevails amongst some of the executive members of District Committees a want of grasp of the principles for which the Society exists, and a want of enthusiasm for their fulfilment. There was general agreement, for instance, amongst those who attended the Conference, that almost all those who join the Society do so in the first instance for the sake of its relief work, and that many never get beyond that stage. 'General business' involving the discussion of principles, aroused only a languid interest at District Committees, and the discussion was as a rule confined to one or two members of the Committee. This want of interest in principles was not confined to the new recruits only, but extended itself even to those who had been working for the Society for a considerable period.

The great development of the casework of the Society of late years has evidently become a new danger in this respect. It has naturally a more concrete and direct personal interest than the advocacy of principles, and as all experience shows, may easily monopolize the whole time and attention of a band of workers necessarily limited. The question does not, of course, come within the scope of the inquiry of this Committee except in so far as the subject of training is concerned, and therefore the Committee would merely emphasize in passing the essential importance of inculcating principles as early as possible in the education of a learner, of impressing upon him that casework is mainly to be used as a means of organization, and that the 'improvement of the condition of the poor' as a whole is a much nobler and more far-reaching object than the relief of a certain number of cases of distress.

The details of training were discussed at the Conference at some length. It appeared that the plans for training varied considerably and that by some, indeed, the necessity of method was hardly appreciated at all. To some extent each Committee must work out its own scheme of training. As the trainers differ, so do the learners in capacity and temperament. The point of chief importance is that every Committee should have the question constantly before it, and should keep a constant watch upon the results of its system, whatever it may be.

There are, however, some general principles which apply to education of all kinds upon which all must be agreed, and which must in practice be worked out by everyone in his own way.

It is of the first importance, and it requires the highest gifts of tact, judgment, and ability, to awaken the curiosity and sustain the interest of the learner. It is a matter which probably requires especially delicate handling in charity organization, because those who join District Committees are for the most part men and women of education and intelligence, who have had knowledge and experience of the world, and have already probably made up their minds upon many questions. Everything depends upon the manner in which they are dealt with at the outset. If they are put to odd jobs of letter writing, visiting, and office work, without having any clear perception of the general drift of the work as a whole, one of two things will probably happen: either they will sink into a mere routine, doing possibly useful work, but not the best work of which they are capable, or they will lose their interest and drop out of the Society altogether. If, however, they are trained to realize from the first the possibilities of the Society as an engine of social reform, they will also realize that they may well give to it the best endeavour of which they are capable, and that it well repays sacrifice of time and other occupations.

In all education, again, the chief object should be to draw out of the learner all that is in him rather than to cram him with principles. The word 'training' has a flavour of pedantry about it against which we have to be on our guard, and especially so when dealing with those who are no longer children. It has been said that 'most commonly the authoritie of them that would teach hinders them that would learne', and there can be no doubt that in charity organization, as in other education, the 'authoritie of the teachers' may easily become a hindrance. It may, if too much obtruded, repel the learner from the outset. It is certain, if it is accepted, to deaden his intellectual activity. The best trainer is probably he who treats nothing, not even a question of principle, as a foregone conclusion, but argues out every question upon equal terms with the learner, and treats his doubts and difficulties with respectful consideration. Nothing is so well calculated to sustain the interest as a healthy intellectual competition, and the learner should be led as far as possible to feel his own way through the difficulties of social questions. No one who is only half convinced is ever likely to do the best work for the Society. The 'authoritie of the teacher', in so far as it prevents the learner from thinking for himself and induces him to take upon trust principles which he does not fully understand becomes a real hindrance to growth. 'The scholler should know that that he knoweth and take nothing upon trust.'

*   *   *

Another point of general application which was raised at the Conference was the importance of what may be called progression in training. The learner should be led as soon as possible from the more simple and elementary part of the work to that which is more complex and responsible. He should be made to feel as soon as possible that he must bear his share of responsibility, not only for the work of his own Committee, but for that of the Society as a whole, and be prepared to take his place eventually as a leader in the forces of charitable reform. If a member of a London District Committee, he should be inspired with the ambition of taking his share in the work of the administrative Committees of the Council as well as in that of his own district. In short, in all training ambition should be excited – not a personal ambition, but the ambition of really doing the best work for the improvement of the condition of the poor.

*　　*　　*

In conclusion, the Training Committee feel that, as they have already indicated, there is no royal road to training, and their hope for the future is rather based upon the wider interest in the subject which is now being manifested than upon any suggestion which they or anyone else can supply. They believe that the Society as a training Society is as yet in its infancy, and that it is capable of almost boundless development. They believe that if the educational functions of the Society were more fully recognized by the public it would lead to a much wider appreciation of its work and expansion of its influence. They would like to see in the Society the nucleus of a future university for the study of social science, in which all those who undertake philanthropic work should desire to graduate.

METHODS OF TRAINING[3]

BY

HELEN BOSANQUET

THE idea that training is a necessary preliminary to charitable work is essentially a new one, so that perhaps it is no
wonder if we are still seeking after the best methods. It is a
search, moreover, that we shall never complete, for, as in
all education, new results and new conditions will bring
new suggestions as to the best way of handling them. But
though we cannot lay down a complete system of rules for
the making of a philanthropist, it is useful from time to
time to survey our experience, to gather together the ideas
which have been found fruitful in the past, and to provoke
both criticism for our present methods and suggestions for
new ones.

And first we may notice that the mere recognition of the
fact that a period of probation and training is necessary is
in itself an important step in that training. For it means, or
should mean, that the novice will begin in the position of a
student; he will take up the work gradually, and will work
at first more with a view to his own education than to the
actual results of his work. I should like to lay stress on this
point, for there is an opposite method which holds that the
right way to train a worker is to immerse him immediately
in the full flood of whatever is going on, and let him sink

[3] Presented to the Council of the Charity Organisation Society in
1900 and printed in the *C.O.S. Occasional Papers* - Third Series -
Paper No. 3.

or swim as the case may be. In one of our London offices ten years ago the method was that said to be practised by some hospitals upon their probationers; during the first few weeks as much work as possible was put on to the novice with a view to testing whether he could stand the strain or whether he would break down under it; if he survived he was then allowed to take his own line and learn what he could, which might be much or little according to his power of observation and asking questions. It was not altogether a bad method; but it was rough and ready, and perhaps rather dangerous in several ways. It is very difficult for the worker trained on these lines to get hold of any general outlook upon the problems he is handling. Sensible ideas he may get in a kind of way by dint of seeing cases classified and treated on fairly consistent lines; but he will tend to work by dead rule instead of by living principles if he has never had leisure to escape from details.

The beginner, then, in any branch of work should be definitely a student, and not an additional office-boy. That does not mean, of course, that he is never to do anything useful; but it does mean that he is to approach the work from an entirely different point of view. We don't want the office-boy to ask the reason why, whenever he is told off to a piece of work; but the merit of the student will probably be proportionate to the number of questions he is capable of asking and the amount of time he gives to understanding what he is doing. In a busy office the temptation for those in authority to lose this point of view is great; we tend to welcome the active, energetic person who likes running about the district on his bicycle, and enjoys nothing so much as making a dozen disconnected inquiries on a dozen different cases which just need completing for committee. Compared with him, the person who is always raising difficulties and asking explanations is very troublesome, and hardly less so the person who sits for hours puzzling himself and others over one set of case-papers.

But thinking is not always waste of time; and the student who is neither thinking nor asking questions may do an immense amount of miscellaneous work without getting much further in understanding. If he is to be properly trained he must be made, at whatever cost of time and trouble, to restrain his enthusiasm for doing and overcome his reluctance to think. He must be made to see that the past has its lessons to teach, the future its dangers to be averted; and above all he must be brought to realize that the present problem before him is not confined to the little room where A and B are wrestling with their fate, but that their trouble is only one aspect, or phase, or point in movements affecting the whole community.

It may be difficult enough to get our student to enter into these wider views, and all the more from the difficulty we shall have in understanding his own attitude. If we could get inside his mind and see what was going on there it would be easier. Sometimes we should find mere ignorance, and that is far from being the most hopeless state. Most of us have been ignorant when we first came to the work; but given the will to learn and a good teacher, ignorance may soon be changed into knowledge. More difficult to cope with is the common prejudice against reading or learning of any kind. 'There is too much real work to be done,' one will say; 'I have no time for your books and theories.' It is very hard to make any headway against such a prejudice as this; to show the student that what we aim at is to make him more and not less practical. His mind is apt to be of the type which thinks nothing real unless he can touch it with his fingers; for him the past is a myth and the future a dream, and the events of today without either causes or consequences. We have no chance with him unless we can exert authority to make him assume the attitude of a student in the hope that the spirit will come later.

A milder form of this prejudice is in the mind of the student who wants to devote himself to one branch of work without knowing anything of others. 'I don't want to read about the poor law,' he will explain; 'it's not the kind of work that I care about.' But though this is an age of specialization, the student must be made to see that he cannot afford to neglect any of the influences affecting the lives in which he is interested: that specialization indeed means learning more, not less. A man is not a specialist because he knows only one thing, but because he knows one thing better than others.

The mind that comes prejudiced in favour of, or against, some particular mode of dealing with its problems will be easier to deal with, just because it has probably grasped the idea of social causation, and will be capable of learning from experience when brought face to face with it. I have seen a strong affection for Socialism die quietly out before experience of good case-work on a background of economic history; and we all know how inevitably the prejudice against the C.O.S. disappears before the understanding of its actual work and methods.

It must be borne in mind that our students come to us grown men and women, with their characters and peculiarities largely developed. That being so, can any general method of training be laid down? Only, I think, in its broader outlines, the details of which must be filled in by the skilful and sympathetic teacher with a view to the circumstances of each case.

Perhaps the first step might always be to find out whether the student really knows what he is aiming at, what it is that he wants to do in taking up charitable work. Often we shall find a mere vague wish to do good, to be of some use to those who seem less fortunate than the average; and then it will be our business to see that this vague aspiration gets its proper object, and becomes a definite desire to promote definite ends. The student must be taught what the good is that he wishes to do, before he can be taught how to do it. Sometimes, on the other hand, we shall find his mind occupied with the very definite but narrow desire of alms-giving, of bringing relief to as many poor people as possible; and by showing him that what he really wants is to make happy and prosperous lives, we shall be able to lead him to wider views and better methods. But almost without exception we shall find it necessary, whether the student's aims are vague or only narrow, to show him that the true end and aim of our work is to get rid of poverty and pauperism altogether, and to raise our people into independence. For the one thing which never seems to occur to the charitable worker is, that his work may be anything finer and more hopeful than making the best of a bad job; that it may have a really regenerating influence.

The first step, then, is to make the student realize more fully and more definitely the issues involved in the work he is undertaking, to know more clearly what he wants, and to want higher things. The next, I suppose, is to help him to find the best ways of achieving his ends; and here comes in the absolute necessity of studying the experience of others. This must be done largely by reading, for experience is history and our only means of making the past our own is by the written word, except in the rare cases where we meet those who have themselves been makers of history. We have, of course, lectures, which we hope are useful in guiding the work of the student; but lectures are very apt to trickle off the mind and leave nothing but vague impressions, unless they are enforced by the harder discipline of reading. To know the history of the English Poor Law, at least in its broader outlines; to have mastered in detail the changes wrought by wise administration in one or two typical parishes; and to have studied the effects of dole charities upon the unfortunate recipients; this, I think, is the minimum which a wise student should allow himself.

It is in some such way as this that one first begins to have a notion of a district as a whole, and to see how all within it are apt to stand or fall together. But this notion of a district as a unity might be made more definite and practical by a study of the particular district in which the student is working, together with its institutions. For our purpose it is generally the Poor Law Union which forms the important area, as being more or less governed with one policy with respect to the treatment of the poor. We must be prepared here to meet with blank ignorance on the part of the student, who has very probably never before come into relation with the life of the people and the institutions affecting it. He may have to learn from the beginning the part played in our social economy by trade unions, friendly societies, guardians and vestrymen; relieving officers and sanitary inspectors will be a new order of beings for him, and the Church will acquire a different significance, when he learns that its influence is not confined to the spiritual side of life. I would urge that a considerable part of his time should be devoted to exploring his Union as if he were Nansen looking for the North Pole. He should take a map, and mark first the limits of the Poor Law Union, with its dismal centre in the workhouse; within those limits he should mark again the different Church parishes, and as he does so learn something of the policy and influence of the Church within those parishes. If he sets himself to hunt down all the numerous philanthropic agencies within the district his work will not only be educational for himself, but may be made of permanent use for others and the basis of real organization in the future. And even if he himself moves elsewhere when his training is over, he will never again be content to work in happy ignorance of his surroundings.

I shall say little of case work, which in one sense is the most important element in training. For one reason, we already have printed papers by experienced trainers on the subject.[4] For another, when the student begins to take up

----

[4] There are a number of papers on 'case work' in various issues of the *Charity Organisation Review* about this time (1900-01).

case work he necessarily abandons more or less the attitude of the student. His work can no longer be directed solely with a view to his own education: whatever is done must be done with a single eye to the necessities of good work, and no experimental bungling can be allowed which may mar that work. I wonder whether we make quite as much use as we might of past cases in this respect. Old case-papers may be tedious to work through, but they are very instructive; and every office might have its dozen or so of illustrative cases for newcomers to study in their early days, including of course, some in which mistakes have led to failure. Other people's mistakes are almost as instructive as our own, and perhaps easier to see. Perhaps the principle on which I should like to lay most stress with reference to training in case work, is that we keep the student from falling into anything like conventionality. Conventional ways of classifying cases, conventional modes of help, conventional rules for making inquiries, all are dangerous, and especially dangerous in our work. It is comparatively easy to learn the little list of categories: *Not likely to benefit, Left to Clergy, Poor Law case, Necessary information refused*, and to class our case under it; what is more important and difficult is to learn how to keep it out of one of these classes, and this requires an insight to which every case is unique and individual. It is easy again to have at one's fingertips the accepted modes of relief; but to plan a scheme by which to raise a family to independence, to construct a raft for the shipwrecked applicant, out of a few shreds of character remaining to him, and steer him safely to solid ground – this is work in which no conventional tradition will help. It requires faculties which are perhaps not present in all our students, but which may be largely developed by a training which insists upon their exercising all their intelligence in devising plans.

We talk a great deal in our work about the necessity of plans. Really the student has to learn to combine two plans

– the one of helping the individual case, the other of raising the district to which it belongs. It is less difficult than it seems at first, for the contradiction which sometimes appears between the two is only apparent, or at most temporary. Moreover, it is a difficulty which all artists have to solve, that of developing both the part and the whole without sacrificing either, in order to attain harmony. I say all artists, for there is always something of the artist about the true philanthropist, and the harmony of life which he aims at creating is hardly less important than that of the painter, the poet, or musician.

APPENDIX II

Economic Teaching at the Universities in Relation to Public well-being.[1]

BY

PROFESSOR A. MARSHALL

THE honour which you have done me in asking me to open a discussion on 'Economic Teaching at the Universities in Relation to Public Well-being' may, perhaps, have arisen from my sending to Mr Loch a 'Plea for the Creation of a Curriculum in Economics and Associated Branches of Political Science in Cambridge'. It was largely occupied with questions of internal organization, on which – like every other ancient corporation – we are jealous of interference, and even of counsel from outside. And on those questions it would be neither right nor expedient that I should speak today.

But, in addition to these matters of private concern, two broad issues were raised in which the public is directly concerned, and which touch very close on the heart of the work of this Committee. The first is: What is the national interest in the supply of trained economists? or, to put the point more definitely, in the supply of persons who give their lives and energies from early manhood upwards to a

[1] A paper presented at a Conference of the Committee on Social Education of the C.O.S. on October 24, 1902, and printed in the *Charity Organisation Review* for January, 1903.

study of economics of the same order and quality as that which is given by professional physicists, physiologists or engineers to their studies? The number of such people is large in every Western land except this; although this is the home of those classical economic writings on which – partially obsolete as they are now – other lands have based their economic knowledge.

The second of the two questions is: How does the study of economics serve as a preparation for business and for public responsibilities?

These two questions together run up into that which I am invited to open today; and perhaps I may be excused for incorporating a few passages from my Plea in the tentative answer which I am to submit – not without some trepidation – as a basis for discussion.

I will, then, begin by looking at some of the causes which are rendering the study of the broad problems of public and private business more urgent than it used to be, and at the same time more suitable for being treated by aid of an academic study of the experiences of the modern world. Of course such a study cannot supersede the need for practical power, instincts, and sympathies which can be trained only by the experience of business and of social life, but it may supplement them. And the first question I would ask is: Has not this training a large part to play in supplementing those practical powers, instincts, and sympathies which can be developed only in action, only through experience? Are not the changes of the present age making it ever more urgent?

First among these changes is the rapid growth of international relations, rising out of the increase of wealth and the developments of telegraphic and other modern means of communication. This growth has made every country more sensitive to the economic movements of its neighbours; and the term 'neighbours' is ever obtaining a wider significance, partly as a result of expansion of empires across the ocean until their frontiers march together in all quarters of the globe. Peace and war have long been governed mainly by the prevailing opinions, true or false, as to national interests and international rivalries in distant fields of commerce, actual and potential. But it is only recently that dependence on distant sources of supply for food and raw produce has made England's continued existence depend on her keeping pace with the forward economic movement of nations against whom she may need to measure her force. In fact England is not, and probably never again will be, completely mistress of her own house. She is not free to weigh the true benefits of a higher culture or a more leisurely life against the material gains of increased economic vigour, without reference to the rate at which the sinews of war are growing elsewhere.

Again, it must be remembered that economic movements are never an isolated series, but are always part of broader movements, in which social and political developments take a leading part; and therefore some general acquaintance with the social and political developments of the leading countries of the Western world is essential for a real, as distinguished from a merely hypothetical, study of the most important of modern economic problems. And this study of recent history is not likely to be carried through except at a University.

Next, the size of the business unit is increasing in every direction; this is so loudly said just now by the man in the street that instances are superfluous. In consequence, the area of economic problems within a country is being enlarged; and financial magnates of one country control some business affairs in others.

This expansion intensifies many social problems and the human aspects of economics generally, especially labour problems; and it raises questions too large for anyone to study satisfactorily in the midst of hurried affairs, unless he has had his attention turned to them before that hurry begins.

A generation or two ago business was relatively simple. Quick wits, prompt energy, and the training of the workshop or counting-house went fairly well by themselves: there was relatively little need for that broad outlook and that versatility of mind which it is the special province of a University to train. But now, while those in subordinate ranks of business often may be content with a narrow outlook, and may need a technical education which it is not the proper function of Universities, or at all events not of the older Universities, to give; that broader training is just what is needed by the higher and more responsible ranks of business, both private and public. For, while the work of subordinates is becoming more specialized, that of our leaders in action is becoming broader and less specialized.

Success in large training has always needed breadth of view.

But both this Committee and economists generally are more nearly concerned with the social and personal elements of human well-being than with the material; and here they come into specially close contact with the strong business man who is also an employer of labour. His material as well as his personal success depends largely on his understanding the real life of the people. His primary relations with his workmen lie indeed in the exchange of pay for labour. But he is likely to fall short even as profit-winner, and he certainly cannot be a good citizen, unless he has thought and cared much about those sides of his workpeople's life and character which are, at most, indirectly reflected in the wages bargain. To learn this from personal contact is ever more difficult for the large employer: he is separated from the mass of the workers by too many strata of subordinates. But broad, modern economic studies will have prepared him to look at the problems of employment from the point of view of the employee as carefully as from that of the employer. Experience shows that this training helps him to see the drift of the complaints urged by his men, and to make concessions quickly and cordially to such as are reasonable. And especially will this be the case if he has combined with his studies that social training which is afforded by the life of a residentiary University of the Anglo-Saxon type.

For such a life draws out the faculties which are needed in the social relations of those who have to deal with large bodies of men and large public interests. On the river and in the football field the student learns to bear and to forbear, to obey and to command. Constant discussion sharpens his wits; it makes him ready and resourceful; it helps him to enter into the points of view of others, and to explain his own; and it trains his sense of proportion as regards things and movements and persons, and especially as regards himself.

Nearly the same preparation for their future responsibilities is needed by those who, as public officials, as ministers of religion, as the owners of land or cottage property, or in any other private capacity will be largely concerned with 'the condition of the people question', with public and private charity, with co-operation and other methods of self-help, and with harmonies and discords between different industrial classes, and with the problems of conciliation and arbitration of industrial conflicts which are ever assuming larger proportions. Those who are nearest to these conflicts can seldom be perfectly impartial arbitrators; and there is here a special call for men who have received a sound training in economics and in political science, and can bring to bear that elasticity of mind and that quickness of sympathy with aspirations and ideals that are not their own which it is the privilege of a residentiary University to foster.

The present age is indeed a very critical one, full of hope but also of anxiety. Economic and social forces capable of being turned to good account were never so strong as now; but they have seldom been so uncertain in their operation. Especially is this true of the rapid growth of the power and inclination of the working classes to use political and semi-political machinery for the regulation of industry. That may be a great good if well guided. But it may work grave injury to them, as well as to the rest of the nation, if guided by unscrupulous and ambitious men, or even by unselfish enthusiasts with narrow range of vision. Such persons have the field too much to themselves. There is need for a larger number of sympathetic students, who have studied working-class problems in a scientific spirit; and who, in later years, when their knowledge of life is deeper, and their sense of proportion is more disciplined, will be qualified to go to the root of the urgent social issues of their day, and to lay bare the ultimate as well as the immediate results of plausible proposals for social reform.

For instance, partly under English influence, some Australasian Colonies are making bold ventures, which hold out special promise of greater immediate comfort and ease to the workers. But very little study of these schemes has been made of the same kind, or even by the same order of minds as are applied to judging a new design for a battleship with reference to her stability in bad weather, and yet the risks taken are much graver. Australasia has indeed a large reserve of borrowing power in her vast landed property, and should the proposed short cuts issue in some industrial decadence, the fall may be slight and temporary. But it is already being urged that England should move on similar lines, and a fall for her would be more serious.

We need, then, to watch more carefully the reciprocal influences which character and earnings, methods of employment and habits of expenditure exert on one another. We need to see how the efficiency of a nation is affected by and affects the confidences and affections which hold together the members of each economic group – the family, employers, and employees in the same business, citizens of the same country. We need to analyse the good and evil that are mingled in the individual unselfishness and the class selfishness of professional etiquette and of Trade Union customs. We need to study how growing wealth and opportunities may best be turned to account for the true well-being of the present and coming generations.

For this work are required the three great faculties – first, perception and observation; secondly, imagination; thirdly, reasoning. None of these can be exercised at all without involving the exercise of the other two. But they are different. Perception must be trained in childhood; the springs of imagination belong to youth; clear reasoning in complex problems comes only with the mature strength of years. Of all these imagination is the greatest. It is imagination which makes the great soldier as well as the great artist, the great business man, and the student who extends the boundaries of science.

Every science requires and trains in various degrees these three faculties – perception, imagination, reason; the use of these three constitutes the centre of the intellectual life of every University. But perhaps there is no science which requires all three in more even proportions than economics; none, therefore, which more properly is of University rank. And in addition, economic studies train the sympathies together with the intellect. This task, which truly belongs to the University, is most excellently performed in its social life, but not equally well in its studies.

But to return to imagination, the greatest of all intellectual faculties. The economist needs it above all, to put him on the track of those causes of events which are remote or lie below the surface, and of those effects of causes which are remote or lie below the surface. For, according to one of those few classical doctrines which has lost none of its force with time, those economic causes and effects which are not seen by the hasty observer are seldom as important as those which are not seen till tracked out by the aid of the scientific imagination.

In smaller matters, indeed, simple experience will suggest the unseen. Charity Organisation Society work, for instance, puts people in the way of looking for the harm to strength of character and to family life that comes from ill-considered aid to the thriftless; even though what is seen on the surface is almost sheer gain.

But greater effort, a larger range of view, a more powerful exercise of the imagination are needed in tracking the true results of, for instance, many plausible schemes for increasing steadiness of employment. For that purpose it is necessary to have learnt how all the economic world is one organic whole; how closely connected are changes in credit, in domestic trade, in foreign trade competition, in harvests, in prices, and how all of these affect steadiness of employment for good and for evil. It is necessary to watch how almost every considerable economic change in any part of the Western world affects employment in some trades at least in almost every other part. It is necessary, not merely to look at those causes of unemployment which are near at hand, but at those which are far off. If we deal only with those that are near, we are likely to make no good cure of the evils we see; and we are likely to cause evils, that we do not see.

Or, to take another example, when by a 'standard rule' or otherwise it is proposed to keep wages high in any trade, the effects on the surface may be pleasant. But imagination set agoing will try to track the lives of those who are prevented by the standard rule from doing work, of which they are capable, at a price that people are willing to pay for it. Are they pushed up, or are they pushed down? If some are pushed up and some pushed down, as commonly happens, is it the many that are pushed up and the few that are pushed down, or the other way about? If we look at surface results, we may suppose that it is the many who are pushed up. But if, by the scientific use of the imagination we think out all the ways in which prohibitions, whether on Trade Union authority or any other, prevent people from doing their best and earning their best, we shall often conclude that it is the few that have been pushed up and the many that have been pushed down.

Experience and a quick wit are needed also. But strong, large habits of scientific use of the imagination can best be formed by University training in the glorious years of the leisure of youth before experience comes; though in London especially there are many who can afford time for it even in their later years.

Again, the generous thoughts of a University, especially when aided by the social training of Oxford and Cambridge, strengthen that use of the imagination which says to a man – put yourself in his place. Especially they help one social class to look at things from the point of view of another social class. And it has been found by experience in England and in America that the young man who has studied both sides of labour questions in the frank and impartial atmosphere of a great University is often able to throw himself into the point of view of the working man and to act as interpreter between them and persons of his own class with larger experience than his own. This is of special importance now that power has passed into the hands of the working classes. The well-to-do may say wise things effectively; but the only class that is strong enough to do wise things that are difficult is the working class.

If we are to get the good without the evil of the modern movements for better housing, for aiding and for disciplining the residium, for municipal efforts for public well-being, and so on, we must have the best minds and characters among the working class on our side. To that end we need two things beyond all others; one is the sympathetic use of the imagination, the other is its scientific use; therefore we not only want practical experience and close contact with reality; we want also that alertness and breadth of mind which are fostered in a greater or less degree by all those studies that are truly of University rank, but by none more than those very studies which directly bear on the industrial efficiency of the social organism; and which direct attention to the ever-widening horizon which our ceaseless victories over nature are opening out for the higher life, not only of the fortunate few, but also of the great mass of the people.

Greek thought and Greek action, political and social, were indissolubly welded together. But English action has been largely separated from English thought. This did, indeed, relatively little harm while English action was chiefly given to bringing into subjection uncivilized races beyond the oceans, and to developing industries which were strong, but insular and crude. But it is doing untold harm now that the Western world is in effect one, now that some other nations are in certain respects marching quicker and are more alert than we, and now that social and economical problems are becoming every day more urgent, partly because our growing wealth and knowledge is every day increasing our responsibilities. All hail, then, to the Committee on Social Education, which is to combine social thought and action in a modern temper, but in due subordination to the great Greek doctrine that the Ideal is that which is most truly Real!

APPENDIX III

EXTRACTS FROM THE CONFIDENTIAL REPORT OF THE SOCIAL EDUCATION COMMITTEE OF THE C.O.S., SUBMITTED JUNE 8, 1903[1]

Proposed two years' course

In order to set before the Members of the General Committee as exactly as possible the characteristics of a course which they think would meet the conditions of the reference, as combining lectures and teaching with practical work in the case of students who look forward to fulfilling official duties or serving on Public Bodies or undertaking special investigations in social science, the Committee have carefully drawn up one typical synopsis, and they would draw attention to certain distinctive features in it.

(1) It assumes a standard of work and intelligence such as might be expected from honour and the better pass students at Universities.

(2) It aims at giving a wide and adequate basis for social theory. It takes for granted that a just and well-understood conception of society is a necessary preliminary to good administrative work.

(3) It touches on the various sides of social science and obligation – the development of society, social economics, some of the problems of social psychology and ethics, such as the formation of individual and social habit, etc.

[1] Attached to the *Minutes of the Council* of the Charity Organisation Society, June 8, 1903.

(4) It includes the history of the development of the industrial classes.

(5) It includes also the history and methods of Poor Law relief and charity, especially during the last three centuries.

(6) It will be noted that it begins in the first year by lectures on 'principles directly bearing upon practice', 'concurrently with some practical work'. It starts indeed from the concrete and the practical, and all through keeps in close relation with it.

(7) Also to supplement the course on the practical side other courses to be given at District Committees and other suitable centres bearing definitely on family and individual life, methods of assistance, and the general organization of aid and relief are set down (see pp. 21 f). These must be read into this typical synopsis as illustrating the practical work which would be required of students.

(8) The course contains much that should probably have been read by students at the Universities. So far as this was the case, it would be modified to meet the actual need of students.

On this typical course two or three criticisms may be made. It may be said that it is not sociological enough. The criticism is in a great measure right; to give a more sociological character some books might be substituted for a few of those on the list. For that purpose, or in connection with a separate set of lectures for which there would probably be ample room and which might be more definitely sociological other such books might be suggested.

Another criticism may be that it should refer less to the 'structure of society' and to 'economic principles' generally, and should be confined chiefly to the study of industrial life and its conditions and to practical administration. In this case again, while lectures and books which furnish teaching on this point are suggested, undoubtedly some useful books might be added, or a course of a limited character, touching very shortly on social theory and development, and dealing at length with industrial conditions and practical work, might be set on foot.

Suggested two years' course

The two years' course which they suggest is for students who are also engaged in practical work (probably as beginners). It is arranged on the principle that, as practical work at once raises the questions of the theory and methods of relief, of the structure and basis of society, and of the economic laws of the industrial world, so the course of study must combine these three departments and treat them simultaneously, proceeding from the less to the more difficult.

Thus in section (a) the student begins with the simpler principles of charitable relief, leading on to the Poor Law, and to public assistance generally, and ending with a special study of systems and conditions.

In section (b) the student begins by raising and considering the fundamental conditions of the existence of society in any form, and works from these historically to the theory of the modern state in its various aspects.

In section (c) the student begins with the general principles of economics, and works from these to special questions of the day (especially Distribution and Wages and State Interference), ending with the consideration of orthodox theories in relation to present conditions.

NOTE: This course is divided into four parts, to occupy about six months each. From some of the books set down selections only would be read.

First Year: Course of study to be followed concurrently with some practical work.

I.   (a) Principles directly bearing upon practice. (Lectures)
         Books: Miss Octavia Hill's 'Homes of the London

Poor', etc. Mrs Bosanquet's 'Rich and Poor', C. S. Loch's 'Charity Organization'.

(b) Theory of the Structure of Society. (Lectures)
Books: Plato's 'Republic', books 1 to 4, with Jowett's 'Introduction'; also Hobbes' 'Leviathan'. (Selections)

(c) Economic Principles
Books: Mill's 'Political Economy'; also Marshall's 'Economics of Industry'.

II. (a) ⎫
    (b) ⎬ As before, with the following additions: –
    (c) ⎭

Under (a) take in the 'History of State Relief of the Poor', with Fowle's 'Poor Law' *or* Mackay's 'Public Relief of the Poor', *or* Aschrott's 'English Poor Law System'.

Under (b) add Nettleship's 'Lectures on Republic'; and essay on Aristotle's 'Conception of the State' (in 'Hellenica'). Take in Aristotle's 'Politics' (books 1 and 2). Rousseau's 'Contrat Social' (books 1 and 2).

Under (c) add parts of Marshall's 'Principles'.

Second Year: (Practical work continuing if possible.)

III. (a) Continue 'History of Poor Law', with Nicholl's and Mackay's 'History', Eden's 'State of the Poor'.
Take in now Local Government, with Chalmers' 'Local Government'.

(b) Continue as before, taking in Theories of the Modern State, with Spencer's 'Study of Sociology', Bagehot's 'Physics and Politics', T. H. Green on 'Freedom of Contract'.

(c) Continue as before, with special attention to modern questions of Distribution and Wages, with parts of Marshall's 'Principles' (as before), Jevons' 'State in Relation to Labour'.

Under (b) and (c) together may now be introduced the questions of the Function of the State (State Interference). Books: Bentham on 'Government', on 'Legislation'; Spencer's 'Man versus the State'.

IV. (During latter half of second year students should probably specialize, taking *either* (a), (b) or (c), *not* all of them.)

(a) Continue History of Poor Law, with (1) Poor Law Provisions in other countries, Reports to Local Government Board, 1875; (2) Special History of Scotland and Ireland; (3) Study of Commissioners' Reports (1817, 1834, 1839, etc.).

Add public provision for assistance and correction, laws relating to children, the sick and imbecile, vagrants, sanitation and housing, education, reformatories.

(b) Bring in now, as a special subject, the Historical Interpretation of Modern State, with Maine's 'Early History of Institutions', Seebohm (selections); also the Philosophical Analysis of Modern State, with Leslie Stephen's 'Ethics', Chapter iii, T. H. Green's 'Principles of Political Obligation', C to G; also the Introduction to Social Psychology, with Stout's 'Analytical Psychology', Chapters v to viii, Tarde's 'Social Laws', 'Les Lois de l'Imitation'.

(c) Introduce History of Economics, with Ingram's 'History of Political Economy', Bagehot's 'Economic Studies', i to iii.

Continue special Study of Wages, with Thorold Rogers' 'Six Centuries of Work and Wages'.

List of supplementary books under the three headings:

(a) First Year.   I. 'C.O.S. Occasional Papers' and series on Special forms of relief; 'Chalmers on Charity' (Masterman's Selections).

II. C. Booth's 'Pictures of Pauperism'; Capper's 'Workhouse System at Great Missenden'.

Second Year. III.

IV. Local Government Board 'Reports', Selections.

(b) First Year. I. Locke's 'Civil Government', More's 'Utopia'.

II. Aristotle's 'Ethics', books viii and ix.

Second Year. III. Seeley's 'Introduction to Political Science' Mill's 'Representative Government'; 'Liberty'.

IV. (1) Tylor's 'Primitive Culture'; also Bryce's 'American Constitution'.

(2) Giddings' 'Elements of Sociology' (part); Bosanquet's 'Philosophical Theory of the State'.

(3) James's 'Psychology' (on the Emotions); Munsterberg's 'Psychology and Life'; Le Bon's 'Psychology of Peoples'.

(c) First Year. I. Adam Smith's 'Wealth of Nations' (part).

II. Walker's 'Political Economy'; Sidgwick's 'Political Economy' (part).

III. Walker's 'Wages'; Cannan's 'Production and Distribution'.

IV. Cliffe Leslie's 'Essays in Political and Moral Philosophy' (Nos. x, xii, xiv); Leslie Stephen's 'Social Rights and Duties' (ii, iii, iv, v in Vol. I); (also parts of Roscher's 'Marx'); and for special study of wages, Booth's 'Life and Labour'.

2. The Course proposed by the Rev C. F. Rogers to deal more directly with conditions of industrial life, from

the Report of the Committee on Social Education, June 8, 1903.

In the first year, students might commence with a sketch of the development of society, and then pass to the History of Labour and the outlines of Economic History; these might be studied in such books as 'The Growth of English Industry and Commerce' (W. Cunningham), 'Six Chapters on Work and Wages' (J. E. Thorold Rogers), 'The Industrial Revolution' (A. Toynbee), and perhaps the historical chapters of Karl Marx's 'Das Kapital'.

Then they might pass to the consideration of the present conditions of life and labour, and to the outlines of economic theory, studying such books as Professor Marshall's 'Economics of Industry', and parts of 'Life and Labour of the People', by Mr Charles Booth.

This would form the first part of the first year's study. Speaking generally it would deal with the normal condition of the industrial classes.

The second part would deal more particularly with the development of social duty, the history of Poor Relief and of charity, of remedial measures generally, whether legislative or voluntary and philanthropic.

Some of the books mentioned above (pp. 15 f.) might be used in connection with this course – 'History of the English Poor Law' (Nicholls and Mackay), 'Charity and Charities' (article in the British Encyclopaedia), etc.

Again, the same question – remedial measures, in relation to legal, charitable, and other agencies – might be treated from the point of view of present conditions considered in relation to immediate remedies. In this regard such works as 'Rich and Poor' (Mrs Bosanquet), 'The Introduction to the Charities Register and Digest', 'The Better Administration of the Poor Law' (Sir W. Chance) might be read.

In the second year the subject might be treated in detail, thus:

a. The family and organization.

(The family as the unit of social life; relation of legal, charitable, and other agencies to one another; sanitary, law, housing, charity organisation, the relation of social work to religious organizations, etc.)

b. The child.

(Education law, underfeeding, industrial questions, under the Poor Law, defective homes, sick, crippled, social improvement, holidays, etc., etc.)

c. The adult.

(Destitution, vagrancy, lunatic, defective, criminal, distressed sick, convalescence, thrift, friendly societies, etc., etc.)

d. Women and the aged.

(Widows, rescue work, the aged under the Poor Law, pension schemes, incurables, etc., etc.)

For this course of study of the subject in detail special monographs on the several questions might be written. There is considerable scope for original work here.

A course of practical work arranged in connection with a District Committee of the Charity Organisation Society would be carried on parallel to this course of lectures and reading on lines similar to those suggested below by Mrs Bernard Bosanquet and Miss Sewell.

*   *   *

Again, if as suggested on p. 77 the lectures were made more definitely sociological, the following books, amongst others, might be used as bearing on different sides of social science : –

Geographical : 'Les grandes routes des peuples; comment la route cree le type social' (Edmond Demolins); Politische Geographie (Friedrich Ratzel).

Historical : History of Intellectual Development, on the lines of modern Evolution (John Beattie Crozier); History of the Philosophy of History (Robert Flint); Die Philosophie der Geschichte als Sociologie (Paul Barth).

Biological: Inquiries into Human Faculty and its Development (Francis Galton); Le Transformisme Social (G. De Greef).

Anthropological: Ueber die Form der Familie (Grosse).

Economic: De la division du travail social (Emile Durkheim); Theory of the Leisure Class (T. Veblen).

Psychologic or Psychologic-ethic: Volker-Psychologie (Wilhelm Max Wundt); Mind in Evolution (L. T. Hobhouse); The Origins of Art (Yrjo Hirn); Ueber sociale Differenzierung (G. Simmel); Social and Ethical Interpretations in Mental Development (James Mark Baldwin); Social Control (Ross).

Ethical: L'Ethique (E. De Roberty); Origin and Growth of the Moral Instinct (Alex. Sutherland).

Philosophical: Microcosmus (R. Hermann Lotze); Introduction to Social Philosophy (John S. Mackenzie).

In regard to attempts at *systematization* the following may be suggested: Principles of Sociology (Herbert Spencer); Dynamic Sociology; or Applied Social Science (Lester Frank Ward); Die Sociologische Erkenntniss (Ratzenhofer).

*　　*　　*

3. Miss Sewell's proposals for practical work:
   (a) Three months should be spent in daily (5 days a week) work at a C.O.S. office, under special guidance. The Secretary to discuss certain definite economic and relief problems in connection with actual cases, and to organize expeditions to the various institutions used in the relief work. (See below, 'Practical Work and its Lessons in a C.O.S. Office'.) No lectures necessarily given in this term.
   (b) A second term should be given to the study of the Poor Law and observation of its working in one or

more Poor Law Unions. This may, or may not, be in connection with the C.O.S. Office.

(c) The rest of the year should be spent over Local Government and the study of normal industrial and social conditions and institutions, together with some definite work under an experienced person in some branch or other of charitable work that is not primarily relief work, e.g.:

The Management of House Property.

The Apprenticing of Children.

Work of School Managers, with which would be connected: School Banks. School Clubs. Country Holidays. School Relief.

District Visiting, where the Visitor is not an almoner.

Evening Clubs and Classes.

The care of Invalid Children.

The care of 'Special', viz. Blind, Deaf, Deficient Children (in connection with School Board Classes).

Collecting and other Savings Banks. Friendly Societies.

Preparation of Returns and Statements, Account-keeping for Charities.

*   *   *

4. A synopsis of practical work at a Charity Organisation Office drawn up by Mrs Bosanquet: –

A. *Case Work*:

i. Study of case-papers and practice in summarizing history of family from running narrative.

ii. Visiting homes as almoner, etc., formation of standard of what a good home should be.

iii. Inquiry work, (a) by correspondence, (b) viva

voce, from employers, previous addresses, references, etc.

    iv. Interviewing applicants for relief, and eliciting essential facts; visiting the home to supplement and confirm.

    v. Preparing a plan of assistance after consultation with relations, employers, etc., and devising means of carrying out plan.

    vi. Reporting on applications, and advising as to suitable treatment.

B. *District Work*:

    i. Topography of district; map showing situation and boundaries of institutions, e.g. Poor Law offices, churches and chapels, hospitals.

    ii. Visits to these institutions and knowledge of income, policy and officials. Study of charitable agencies in district, including endowed charities.

    iii. Industrial conditions of neighbourhood, with rates of wages in various industries.

    iv. Trade Unions, Friendly Societies, Clubs, etc., and proportion of people influenced.

    v. Policy of Guardians as to Relief, and its effect on district; what people receive Outdoor Relief, how it is supplemented; in what industries are they engaged; how do their earnings compare with those of similar age and sex not receiving.

    vi. Housing and sanitation. Reporting of sanitary defects; study of overcrowding and best means of dispersing the people from congested areas.

C. *Organization*:

    i. Inducing co-operation on sound principles amongst various agencies.

    ii. Organizing meetings, lectures, etc., amongst charitable workers.

iii. Organizing (a) Collecting, savings banks and other thrift-agencies; (b) workers amongst schoolchildren; (c) district nursing, provident dispensaries.

iv. Working on Local Government institutions, e.g. as Poor Law Guardians, County Councillors, etc., or promoting the election of desirable candidates.

Printed and bound by CPI Group (UK) Ltd, Croydon, CR0 4YY

17/10/2024

01775689-0004